ALAN GAUNT

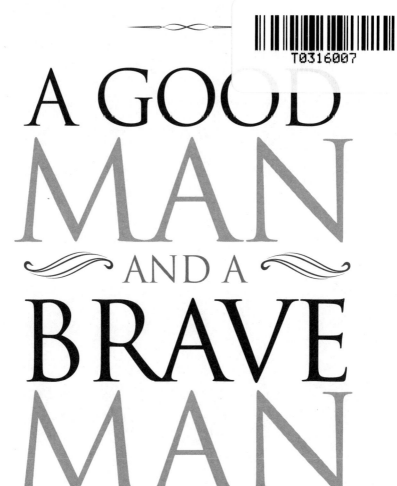

A GOOD MAN AND A BRAVE MAN

THE STORY OF A GLOUCESTERSHIRE SOLDIER,
CECIL THOMAS PACKER, 1885 – 1916

ALAN GAUNT

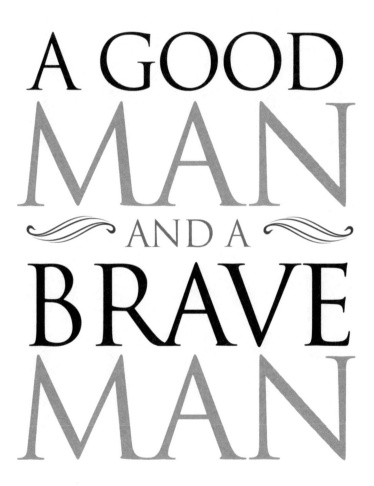

A GOOD MAN AND A BRAVE MAN

THE STORY OF A GLOUCESTERSHIRE SOLDIER,
CECIL THOMAS PACKER, 1885 – 1916

MEREO

Mereo Books

1A The Wool Market Dyer Street Cirencester Gloucestershire GL7 2PR
An imprint of Memoirs Publishing www.mereobooks.com

A Good Man and a Brave Man: 978-1-86151-530-8

First published in Great Britain in 2017
by Mereo Books, an imprint of Memoirs Publishing

Copyright ©2017

Alan Gaunt has asserted his right under the Copyright Designs and Patents Act 1988 to be identified as the author of this work.

A CIP catalogue record for this book is available from the British Library.

The address for Memoirs Publishing Group Limited can be found at
www.memoirspublishing.com

The Memoirs Publishing Group Ltd Reg. No. 7834348

The Memoirs Publishing Group supports both The Forest Stewardship Council® (FSC®) and the PEFC® leading international forest-certification organisations. Our books carrying both the FSC label and the PEFC® and are printed on FSC®-certified paper. FSC® is the only forest-certification scheme supported by the leading environmental organisations including Greenpeace. Our paper procurement policy can be found at www.memoirspublishing.com/environment

Typeset in 12/18pt Century Schoolbook
by Wiltshire Associates Publisher Services Ltd. Printed and bound in Great Britain by Printondemand-Worldwide, Peterborough PE2 6XD

CONTENTS

∽

ACKNOWLEDGEMENTS

There have been so many people who have given generously of their time and contributed with information to help me put together the jigsaw of Cecil's life. I hope I have done those kind people justice with the finished work, and I extend my grateful thanks to them all with inclusion in these acknowledgements.

I must first and foremost record my considerable indebtedness to Jenny Cunningham of Poole Keynes, who is a fount of knowledge concerning the history of the village and who masterminded my visits to that place. She also deserves a huge vote of thanks for her invaluable help with the research on Cecil's time there. Thank you Jenny.

To the family of Dennis Packer, Anne, Maureen, Michael, Kathy and Edward, who shared their family's oral history memories with me.

To Gordon and Pamela Ayres, and to Teresa Smith, who provided valuable information on the subject of shepherding in the village. I am also deeply indebted to the various contributors to the Great War Forum on Chris Baker's website www.long-long-trail.co.uk, who were most helpful in explaining various military matters to me

To Katherine Cole and Darryl Moody at Swindon Local Studies Library, who were most generous with their help and advice. To the staff at Cirencester Library, Gloucestershire Archives and the Wiltshire & Swindon History Centre for their help and guidance. To David Colcombe of Devizes, whose vast knowledge of the GWR opened the door to Cecil's work for that company; and to Swindon's Steam Museum Assistant Curator, Felicity Jones, who kindly added detail to that intelligence.

To Charles Cook of Minety, who provided me with the details of Cecil's early but brief Army service.

To Gordon McKay, who provided his usual wise and helpful comments having read the original draft, and to Gerald Packer, who kindly donated the impeccable contemporary postcard showing Poole Keynes Cross.

To the various villagers of Poole Keynes and Kemble who were so kind and helpful to me: Gill Awdry, June Baker, David Collins, Chris and Diane Fletcher, Bob Hammond, Nancy Legg, Dot Slade, Alan and Margaret Stanford, Mary Timbrell, Richard Tomlin and Ken Wellings.

To Adrian Snow, who supplied the wonderful description of Cecil's cottage in its original condition, and to David Tattersfield of the Western Front Association for kindly providing Cecil's army pension details.

And last but by no means least I must also thank my dear wife Shirley, who has supported, guided and advised me throughout the writing of this book.

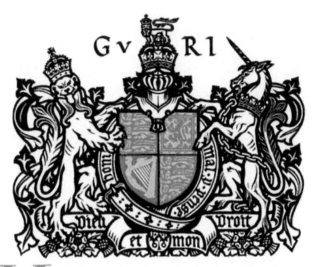

G v R 1

H E whom this scroll commemorates was numbered among those who, at the call of King and Country, left all that was dear to them, endured hardness, faced danger, and finally passed out of the sight of men by the path of duty and self-sacrifice, giving up their own lives that others might live in freedom. Let those who come after see to it that his name be not forgotten.

20550, PRIVATE Cecil Thomas Packer

8th Service Battalion., Gloucestershire Regiment
Died, France & Flanders, 13/12/1916
Born: Minty, Wilts, Enlisted: Cirencester

INTRODUCTION

Cecil Packer was the great-grandfather of my wife, Shirley. We originally knew very little about him apart from the fact that he had died during the First World War and that there was apparently something 'different' about the manner of his death. Curiosity therefore started our research into his life, and our first discovery was that he had been killed 'accidentally' in France while based well away from the front line. Our next discovery was that he had previously served in both the Gallipoli and Somme campaigns, and we were struck by the awful irony that he should be killed by accident at a time when hundreds of thousands of men across the world were deliberately seeking to kill each other every day. It also seemed immensely sad that that he should have survived the horrors of Gallipoli and the slaughter on the Somme only to be killed in an area that was safely away from the bloodshed of the battlefront.

Our enquiries revealed that Cecil was obviously well-regarded, both within his family and the wider community of the village where he lived and worked, so we thought it important that his story should be told. There is nothing grand or fancy about Cecil's upbringing – indeed his childhood has been described as 'very average' – but that's the real importance of his story. It is not the story of a traditional hero in the mould of Nelson or Wellington but that of a village shepherd, a local man who did not come from the nobility or the ranks of the nation's leaders but was simply a man who loved his family and died in the service of his country.

I took the title of this book from a tribute paid to him by an Army comrade in writing to Cecil's widow after he was killed. It is not only a brief but heartfelt tribute to a fallen friend and comrade; it is the summation of a man's life, and a story which I think deserves to be known by a much wider audience.

CHAPTER ONE

EARLY DAYS

Cecil's background was typical of so many in late 19th Century rural England. He was born Cecil Thomas Packer on the 7th July 1885, the fifth child of Thomas and Ellen Packer (formerly Skuse) who lived in the village of Minety (also known as 'Minty') in Wiltshire. The Packers could trace their roots in the village at least as far back as 1677, when Cecil's 5x great-grandfather had been born there. Cecil's older siblings were Alice Lillian (born in 1876); Sarah Florence (born in 1878); Samuel George (born in 1879); and William John (born in 1882). Cecil's birth was registered by his mother, who recorded her husband

1

Thomas's occupation as 'Farm Labourer'. Cecil was baptised in the Minety Parish Church of St Leonard on the 2nd August 1885.

Thomas, Ellen and their five children then moved about four miles away to live in the village of Poole Keynes, which at that time was still in Wiltshire. Fred Thacker, in his contemporary book *The Stripling Thames,* wrote 'Poole Keynes is a tiny community', and indeed it was, consisting simply of 34 dwellings which comprised five farms (Church Farm, Gents Farm, Glebe Farm, Lower Farm & West End Farm) together with their tied cottages, and with a total population of only 129. The village came into Gloucestershire when the county boundary was moved in 1897.

The Poole Keynes Rate Book for the 9th August 1890 records 'Thomas Packer' as a ratepayer living at an address known as 'Old Mill Cottages', which was situated in open countryside to the east of the village. A short while afterwards Cecil's younger brother (Rowland Edward) was born there on the 19th August. However, when the 1891 census was completed on the 5th April, the family, Thomas and Ellen with children Sarah (14), Alice (13), Samuel (11), William (8), Cecil (5) and baby Rowland, had moved on and were shown to be living at number 97 Poole Keynes. This was then one of a pair of cottages close to the village centre and positioned sideways on to the road, while the attached cottage, no. 98 Poole Keynes, was described on the census form as being 'uninhabited'.

Life in this little cottage must have been really cramped for everyone, because it was a very basic one-up one-down property with a small rear wash-house and a privy, or toilet, at the far end of the garden. Water came from a well at the side of no. 98 which was shared with the adjacent cottage, no. 100 Poole Keynes, although that property was yet another described as uninhabited at the time of the census.

No. 97 Poole Keynes was tied to Lower Farm which, with its complex of stone barns, cow byres and coach-house stable, is about 90 yards or so to the south of the cottage and was occupied by farmer William Large, for whom Thomas and Ellen both worked. The farmhouse itself was, and still is, a prominent and imposing building of Cotswold stone under a stone-tiled roof and although much altered over the years, is said to date from the 17th Century.

Thomas and Ellen are shown on the census form, together with their son Samuel George Packer, as being 'Farm Servants'. This is an interesting description because 'farm servants' generally differed from 'farm labourers' in that they were usually engaged for short periods of time (often no longer than a year) rather than being employed on the farm all year round. They also had no set working hours and had to be available whenever required by the farmer, so life cannot have been easy for them.

The arrival of Thomas's family in Poole Keynes saw young Cecil being sent to the local school. This was situated at the edge of the village on the road to Oaksey, where it had been built, with an attached master's house, on part of the front garden for the Rectory. It had opened in 1847 for 35 children but often failed to achieve that number, the 1906 Kelly's Directory recording an average attendance of just 20. The school was finally closed in 1922 and the children were then transported by horse and cart to school in Kemble. The former school building now serves as the Poole Keynes village hall.

The 1901 Census, taken on the 31st March, found the family still living at 97 Poole Keynes, where youngest daughter Clarice Ethel Packer was born in March 1894. Older daughters Alice and Sarah had both married and left home: Alice had married Frederick Stevens in January 1899 and Sarah had wed Ernest Musty in February 1901. Thomas's sons Samuel and William had also moved on and both were working away up in Yorkshire as railway porters.

However Thomas's elderly father, Samuel Packer, had now joined the household. He was an 83-year-old widower and former 'Road Labourer' who had moved to the village from his previous home in Hankerton Road, Minety. Old Samuel lived with Thomas's family until his death on the 8th January 1903. Also staying at No 97, at least on census night, was Thomas's five-year-old niece, Elizabeth Packer, who was born in Malmesbury.

The property next door, no. 98 Poole Keynes, which was empty at the time of the last census, was no longer listed because it had been merged with 97 to provide some much-needed additional accommodation at that address. The 1911 census described no. 97 as having 'four rooms' consisting of a kitchen and sitting room on the ground floor with two bedrooms above; this clearly indicates an increased level of accommodation compared to that which existed in 1891. The original wash-house at the rear and the outside privy were not affected by these changes. Nonetheless, and despite these extra rooms, the house will still have been full to overflowing, with a total of eight occupants ranging in age from five to 83. However that type of circumstance was not uncommon at the time; the bedrooms were probably divided by curtains to afford some degree of privacy, while several children often had to share one bed.

The census also describes Cecil as 'day labourer on farm', meaning that he was simply employed on a day-to-day basis without any permanency of employment, and being a fifteen-year old, he would probably have only been engaged on fairly basic farming work. However the men of the Packer family have all been tall and robust, and Cecil was no exception. He was a sturdy lad and physically well able to do a day labourer's work on the farm. This included such jobs as bird scaring, which was necessary to keep the birds away from freshly-sown seeds, or clearing the stones which blunted the blades of the horse-drawn ploughs. As he became older and gained experience with farm work he graduated to more demanding tasks such as harrowing. The harrow consisted of a heavy frame with iron teeth which was dragged over a freshly-ploughed field by horses to break up the clods of earth, remove weeds and level out the soil ready for the seeds to be sown.

This particular census additionally goes on to describe Cecil's father, fifty-year-old Thomas, as a 'cattleman on farm', a new job which seems to have been something of an improvement on his original role of 'farm servant'. Local resident Ronnie Roe, in an interview before he died in 1999, said that by the 1920s Lower Farm 'probably had 60 milking cows and two men to milk them', and the size of that herd is, in all likelihood, about the same as it was when Thomas worked on the farm – and in all probability doing the milking amongst his various other tasks.

Nonetheless, Thomas's new job does not appear to have resulted in any improvement to his wages or situation generally, because he still needed to apply for charitable relief from the Parish. The poor of the village received payment from 'Henry Poole's Charity Fund', which dated from 1722, having been created under the will of Henry Poole, a local landowner. The will established a fund for the poor in the parishes of Kemble, Oaksey and Poole Keynes which was to be managed in each parish by 'the Minister, Churchwardens and Overseers.' They were instructed that the money should be paid out yearly, with the only proviso being that it should not be given to those already receiving alms. The distribution of the money was left to the discretion of the administrators, who were simply told that it should be shared 'in such proportions as shall seem meet'.

Money was paid out at the beginning of January (typically around the 6th to the 9th) and always took place at 12 noon in the village's schoolroom. The number of families from Poole Keynes receiving their annual 'Poor Money' varied between fifteen and twenty, and the surviving records show that Thomas received regular payments which started in 1891 and continued at least until 1915. The amount he received varied each year and was often dependent upon the number of children that he and Ellen were apparently looking after ('children' were defined as being those under 10 years of age); the highest payment was 4/- in 1895, while the lowest payment was 1/5d in 1909 and 1910. Most of the payments were recorded in the parish's 'Book of Vestry Meetings' although some were simply recorded on scraps of paper tucked inside the book.

Bob Hammond's family have farmed at Lower Farm for many years, and Bob said that the milk from the herd at Poole Keynes always went to Cirencester. In order to reach the town, the milk was taken from the farm in churns for the short two-mile journey by horse and cart to Kemble railway station, where it was loaded aboard the branch line train for the slightly longer five-mile journey to Cirencester. The station at Kemble village is now simply described as 'Kemble', but at that time it was known as 'Kemble Junction' because it also served the seven-and-a-half-mile branch line to Tetbury as well as that to Cirencester. Although much of Cirencester's rail traffic had been concerned with the transportation of goods from the town to markets in places as far afield as Bristol and London, the trains still brought a considerable amount of produce into the town, and milk from Poole Keynes was just one of those commodities.

Upon arrival at the town's station the milk was

taken to the premises of the Cirencester Dairy Company in Ashcroft Road. An advert in the Baily & Woods Cirencester Directory for 1908-1911 announced that the dairy produced: 'High Class Dairy Produce. New and Separated Milk, New Laid Eggs, Devonshire, Dorset and Local Butter, Fresh Cream and Devonshire Clotted Cream. Honey etc'. Somewhat surprisingly I think for a dairy, they also advertised the sale of 'White and Smoked Wiltshire Bacon'. Although the dairy later occupied the building that is now home to the 'Stepping Stones Nursery and Pre-School', its location in the early years of the 20th Century was probably immediately adjacent to Ashcroft Road's junction with Cricklade Street.

Thomas's other tasks will have covered all aspects of the tending and rearing of cattle. These included such jobs as driving them to and from cowsheds and pasture fields, cleaning the cowsheds, attending to the cows at calving time and feeding them in the winter months with roots and cattle cake. Being able to look after a herd of cows successfully was time-consuming work for him which, more often than not, did not end until dusk.

When the day's work was finished, Thomas could walk home to his evening meal prepared by Ellen. For many farm workers at the turn of the 20th century, this would have comprised bacon or pork stew served with vegetables grown in the garden. I don't know if Thomas kept his own pig, but the 1900 OS Map for the village shows the garden of the cottage to have been large enough for him to have done so; and it does show a structure which could well have been the pigsty. If that was the case then Thomas would have had the pig slaughtered by the 'Pig Man' who came from the adjacent village of Oaksey and travelled around the villages in the area for that purpose.

Ronnie said that the cows on the farm were British Shorthorns and described the routine with cows as follows:

'My late mother could milk a cow in a matter of five minutes – strip her right out. You would get about 2½ to 3 gallons from a good milker. After the calving they were rested and not got in calf until they were built up again. They used to leave the calf with the cow about three weeks or a month until they were really a strong calf, and then they were known as a 'weaned off calf'. They were not sent to market until they could eat hay, eat dry food and be completely weaned off milk. You never saw a calf at the market taken straight off the mother then. And of course they made more money – they were veal, you see. Not a nice thought to many people I know, but at least they were a valuable animal. When the cow was to be got in calf again she did come down again in the autumn when milk was at its highest price. They used to rest their animals then.'

Around this time in his life, Cecil seems to have believed that he could find better and more exciting work than simply being a farm labourer. Accordingly, on the 4th February 1904 at the age of 18 years and 6 months, he travelled to Cirencester and joined the Army, enlisting in the Gloucestershire Regiment. Cecil is described on his Army attestation document as being 5 feet 10 inches tall, weighing 159lbs and with a chest expansion from 33½" to 35½". His face has a fresh complexion with grey eyes and brown hair. His 'Certificate of Medical Examination' recorded: 'He can see the required distance with either eye: his heart and lungs are healthy: he has the free use of his joints and limbs, and he declares that he is not subject to fits of any description'.

Cecil was then sent to the Regiment's Depot at Horfield Barracks in Bristol to begin his Army training. The barracks dated from 1847 and had been built to house the 28th (North Gloucestershire) and the 61st (South Gloucestershire) Regiments of Foot after the area had been the scene of serious rioting. The 61st and 28th regiments were then merged in 1881 to form the 1st and 2nd battalions of the Gloucestershire Regiment. The barracks were eventually demolished in 1966. However

Cecil apparently soon discovered that Army life was not to his liking and so on the 31st March 1904, just under two months after he signed on, he was discharged from the Army 'by purchase' in the sum of £10. This was a considerable sum of money that had to be found to secure Cecil's release from the Army because average rural wages at the time, for example, only amounted to around £2 per month.

Shortly afterwards on the 11th April 1904, still seeking to better himself, Cecil obtained a job as a labourer working for the Great Western Railway in Swindon about 17 miles from Poole Keynes. The Swindon Works of the GWR were huge and covered a site of some 326 acres, mostly surrounded by high brick or stone walls. There were a total of 14 entrances to the Works, with each entrance having a gatehouse manned by a watchman who was often a worker who had been injured and moved to lighter duties. It was at one of these manned gatehouses that Cecil and the other workmen signed on and off at the beginnings and ends of their shifts. Although his brief stay with the Army in Bristol will have shown him a wider world than the somewhat enclosed life of a small agricultural village, Cecil must still have felt overpowered by his arrival at this vast and confusing complex.

Cecil's contemporary at the Works, the railway

worker and author Alfred Williams, referred in his book
Life in a Railway Factory to the impact that the works
had on new workmen arriving there. He graphically
described the stark difference between the GWR Works
and the nearby countryside:

'To view it from the interior is like looking around
the inner walls of a fortress. There is no escape for the
eye; nothing but bricks and mortar, iron and steel,
smoke and steam arising. It is ugly; and the sense of
confinement within the prison-like walls of the factory
renders it still more dismal to those who have any
thoughts of the hills and fields beyond.'

Williams also portrayed the reception of a new
worker, writing that he 'attracts considerable attention;
all eyes are immediately fixed upon him. If he is a total
stranger to the place he will be shy and awkward, and
will need careful and sympathetic instruction; it will be
some time before he is entirely used to his surroundings'

Interestingly, Alfred Williams thought highly of
those workmen, such as Cecil, who came to the Works
from a life in the country compared with their fellow-
workers from the town. 'The workmen who come from
the villages,' he wrote, 'are usually better-natured and
also better-tempered than those who are strictly of the
town, although there are exceptions to the rule. On the
whole, however, they make the more congenial mates,

and they work much harder and are more conscientious. The country workman is fresh and tractable, open to receive new ideas and impressions of things... he is very proud of his new situation.'

The locomotive side of the Works was located north of the main London to Bristol railway line and situated primarily between Rodbourne Road and the railway line to Gloucester and Cheltenham. It consisted of numerous workshops of different sizes which manufactured or repaired component parts to be assembled into new or rebuilt locomotives. Each of these workshops was identified by a letter, and it was amongst this enormous array of buildings that Cecil's workshop was located. The rules of the GWR required that the men use the Works entrance nearest to their workplace which, for Cecil, was the Rodbourne Road entrance.

Cecil's particular place of work was the 'L1 Tube Cleaners Shop', and the 1929 layout plan of the railway works shows this workshop to have been located where the Gap fashion store (Unit 58/60) in the North Shopping Mall of the Swindon Designer Outlet Village now stands. Cecil's job, not surprisingly in view of the workshop's title, was cleaning tubes. The barrel of a steam engine boiler contained numerous metal tubes through which the steam passed, and it was in this workshop where those tubes were prepared.

The tubes were firstly cut to the appropriate size and then ground down to fit into the barrel of the engine, some of which took as many as 325. When the cutting and grinding of the tubes was complete, it was Cecil's job to carefully check and clean them, removing any metal debris, burrs and dirt so that the tubes were ready to be installed in the boiler. This aspect of the work was undertaken in the adjacent Boilermakers' Workshop, of which Tim Bryan, a former Keeper of the GWR Museum in Swindon, wrote: 'It is not an understatement to say that the quality of workmanship in the Swindon Boiler Shop was second to none, and it enjoyed a high reputation both inside and outside the company'. This quotation neatly illustrates the fact that, by properly ensuring the cleanliness of the boiler tubes before they could be fitted in the boiler, Cecil was making an important contribution to the esteem in which the Boiler Shop was held.

There are no records to indicate whether Cecil travelled daily from Poole Keynes to his work or whether he took lodgings somewhere in Swindon. However, it is most likely that he lived in lodgings, like the majority of unmarried workmen, because it was generally expected that workers should live close to the Works. This situation was best described by Alfred Williams, who wrote that the Company tended 'to keep out those who do not live in the borough or within a certain area around the town or, if they are given the chance of a start, it is only upon condition that they leave their homes and live under the shadow of the factory walls'. The reason behind this policy was apparently to encourage wages earned in the town to be 'spent there in the payment of rent or the purchase of provisions and clothes.'

The high walls surrounding the railway works gave rise to the local expression 'working inside' to describe the men who worked there, and life 'inside' the works was hard and long, with a working week of 54 hours spread over five and a half days. On Mondays to Fridays the morning shift started at 6.00am and lasted until 8.15am when there was a break for breakfast. The shift resumed at 9.00am before breaking for lunch at 1.00pm. The afternoon shift lasted from 2.00pm until 5.30pm. There was no afternoon shift on Saturdays, while Sundays were completely free. The start and finish of each shift was marked by the sounding of the works hooter, which could be heard all over the town and surrounding countryside. Discipline was strict, and even toilet breaks were controlled; a ticket had to be given to the attendant, and wages would be deducted if the break lasted more than ten minutes.

It was while Cecil was working for the GWR that he

met and fell in love with Florence Annie Davis, one weekend sometime around 1904 to 1906. She was better known as 'Flo' and was the second daughter of Master Stonemason Francis Edward or 'Frank' Davis and Sarah Annie Davis (formerly Harris). The Davis family had originated from the Bisley/Chalford area near Stroud in Gloucestershire, where Frank's father Charles had also been a stonemason. Frank had brought his family to live in Oaksey in about 1886/87 and rented a cottage in Church Farm Road, where Flo was born on the 1st April 1888.

By 1901 Frank and his family had moved to Flintham, just outside the village, before going on to live in Poole Keynes during the late summer or early autumn of 1904. This dating is indicated by a somewhat terse note from the Reverend Benjamin Mallam written in the margin of the Parish Baptism Register on the 18th September. He recorded that the Davis family 'took a cottage in Poole' but that two of Flo's younger brothers, Walter and Stanley, 'were two and four years old but were not baptised' – an omission which the family's new and ever-vigilant vicar promptly rectified.

It has been said that Cecil and Flo were made for each other, and they were certainly well matched; Cecil was by then aged around 19 or 21 and probably not too different in appearance from his military description in the early part of 1904. He was tall and handsome, although by that time he had grown a neatly-trimmed moustache which he later grew into a handlebar shape. His hair was combed with a parting on the left and cut short in the style of the period. Flo, who was just three years younger, was tall like him but fine-boned. She was very attractive, with a good-looking oval face and fair complexion under dark brown hair. Her brown eyes were warm and compassionate above a strong nose and a kind but firm mouth.

They met at a Sunday afternoon village fete in Poole Keynes or possibly Oaksey. Neither village had any public open space, so the fete was held on private land loaned for that purpose; in Oaksey this was in Oaksey Park or in the gardens of the larger landowners, while in Poole Keynes it was either in the extensive gardens of the Rectory or those of the larger farmhouses such as Lower Farm. The annual fete was an important event in the life of the village and much planning went into its organisation. Colourful bunting adorned the trees surrounding the venue and hung around the house in whose grounds the fete was held. Music was provided by one of the various brass bands that flourished in the area, and everyone attending wore their 'Sunday best' clothes.

Fetes in the two villages were markedly similar:

raffle tickets were sold to raise funds, often for the church, and there were various stalls selling all manner of items like cakes, sweets, bric-a-brac, plants, handicrafts and small home-made articles of clothing. There were events such as fancy dress and baking competitions; there were games such as Skittles and 'Splat the Rat' or 'Find the Egg'- a popular local game which involved hiding one whole egg balanced in sawdust and hidden amongst many empty eggshells. There were also races for all ages and a tug-of-war for the men of the village as well as a game called 'Throw the Mangel' or 'Mangold Hurling'. This was an interesting sport which basically involved throwing a root vegetable as far as possible. The game dated from the Middle Ages and was played all over England, but it was particularly associated with the West Country and reached its peak of popularity around this time before dying away during the Second World War. This was on account of the fact that rationing at the time decreed a much better use for the vegetables.

Flo was helping out in the fete's refreshment tent, selling sandwiches, tea and cakes, and customer numbers were undoubtedly boosted, particularly amongst the young men of the village, by her presence as much as by the provision of a good cup of tea and a nice piece of cake. Nonetheless, and despite her evident popularity, it was Cecil who won her heart, and he would prove to be a kind and loving husband.

Following a successful courtship, and with the agreement of both sets of parents, the banns of marriage between Cecil and Flo were read aloud in the Poole Keynes Church. The banns are proclamations of an intended wedding made in the couple's parish church so that anyone who may know of any impediment to the marriage may object. They were read on three successive Sundays before the wedding ceremony could take place. In this case there were clearly no objections. Shortly thereafter, as recorded in the Parish Register, the marriage was duly 'solemnized after Banns' at a ceremony held on Saturday the 28th September 1907 when Cecil was aged 22 and Flo was 19. The witnesses to the marriage were Flo's father Frank, a friend of the couple Mabel Saunders, and Cecil's young sister Clarice Ethel Packer. The Certificate simply describes Cecil as being a 'Labourer' while the box showing Flo's 'rank or profession' is struck through, indicating that she was not engaged in any employment.

By the time that Cecil and Flo's first son, Francis Thomas Packer (or 'Frank'), was born on the 29th June 1908 they were living at 46 Albion Street Swindon, and the Birth Certificate described Cecil's job as a 'Labourer Railway Factory'. Frank's birth was one of more than

1,400 births in Swindon during that year, an increase over the previous year. A report by the Borough's Medical Officer of Health fascinatingly attributed this continued increase in population to the fact that 'the conditions of life are normally such in this town as to favour a high rate of productiveness.'

Albion Street was located in the town's 'Kings Ward', which was described in the same report as being 'favourably situated' and 'a favourite residential locality: its normally low death rate vouches for its salubrity.' Cecil and Flo's house was a terraced property with a small rear garden, located to the south of the Wilts and Berks canal. It was quite modern, having been built in 1895 with brick walls under a slate roof. The accommodation was generous for the time and consisted of a living room, kitchen and scullery on the ground floor with three bedrooms upstairs as well as an outside toilet or 'privy'. Despite the move to Swindon however, family ties with Poole Keynes remained, and Frank was baptised in the village on the 2nd August, Cecil's abode being listed in the Parish Baptism Register as 'Swindon' and his job as a 'Labourer'.

When Cecil started working for the GWR he was on a wage of 10/8d per week, which had risen to 16/6d by 1905, although the records of the GWR do not indicate if his wages were ever subsequently increased. If he and

Flo were renting their house while living in the town, then the rent would probably have been around five shillings to 5/6d per week. Prices at the time were generally stable: bread cost 5½d for a 4lb loaf, Cheddar cheese was 10d per pound, milk 3d a quart, butter 1/4d to two shillings a pound, and a dozen eggs cost between 8d and two shillings. Of the meat that was available, brisket cost 5½d lb, a leg of mutton 9½d lb, chops and belly pork 8d lb; cod was also priced at 8d lb. Of course the rear garden of the house provided scope for Cecil and Flo to grow their own vegetables, such as potatoes and greens.

If Cecil felt that he might be able to afford an evening out at the pub, he could expect to pay something around 2½d for a pint of beer. The Ship in Westcott Place, now closed, was only a short walk from Albion Street, although it was probably then still a place of some notoriety. In 1903 barmaid Esther Hettie Swinford was working in the bar when she was shot dead by her former fiancé, who was executed in Devizes the following year.

Apart from public houses and the many working men's clubs, the other major source of entertainment and recreation in the town was the Mechanics' Institute, of which Cecil was a member by virtue of his employment with the GWR. Built in 1859 in the railway village close to the GWR Works, it was described at the time as 'the only centre of healthy recreation in Swindon.' It housed a large theatre, a well-stocked library and various smaller rooms which were used by Institute members for a whole range of other social, educational and cultural activities. Other benefits arising from Cecil's employment with the GWR were the various 'perks of the job' such as an allocation of coal and subsidised firewood, as well as the free passes and subsidised privilege tickets for train travel.

The first of the town's cinemas was not built until 1910, but another potential source of entertainment for Cecil and Flo, apart from the Mechanics' Institute, was the Empire Theatre. Dating from 1898, the theatre was situated 'in a commanding position' on the corner of Groundwell Road and Clarence Street and had a seating capacity of around 1,500. However visiting the theatre then was apparently not the more sophisticated pastime that it has since become. Writing of the Empire in the early years of the 20th century, a study of the town undertaken by the Burderop Park Training College reported: 'older theatre-goers will remember that the crowds in those days were by no means as orderly and well-behaved as they are today. Queueing was unknown. You just pushed your way to the box office. The weaker were jostled on to the pavement, and broken limbs and ragged tempers were often the result.' The Empire Theatre was demolished in 1959 and replaced by a 1960s office block in which I worked for some nine years.

There was a general acceptance in those days that a job in the GWR Works was 'a job for life'. Alfred Williams wrote, 'once a man becomes settled in the factory he is reluctant to leave it… he usually remains there to the end of his working days', while Rosa Matheson quoted a worker who started as a teenager and said 'once you went in there, you were there for life. I was sixty-four plus when I finished'. Whether this was intended to be the case with Cecil we shall never know, but despite the benefits of a regular and comparatively well-paid job, allied to the advantages of town life in a modern house, Cecil's time with the GWR was to last for only just over four years.

The Swindon Works was notorious for the poor quality of the air, and Alfred Williams argued that much sickness amongst the GWR workers 'may be attributed to the foul air prevailing – the dense smoke and fumes from the oil forges, and the thick, sharp dust and ashes from the coke fires. Colds are exceptionally common, and are another result of the bad atmospheric conditions; as soon as you enter into the smoke and fume you are sure to begin sniffing and sneezing. The black dust and filth is being breathed into the chest and lungs every moment.'

This continual exposure to smoke and fumes gradually had an effect on Cecil's health, and he suffered with chest complaints and breathing difficulties. He had yearned to go back to the clean air of Poole Keynes in order to better his health for some time, but had been thwarted by the lack of jobs and available accommodation. However a vacancy for a shepherd then arose in the village, and the job came with a tied cottage, so, supported by Flo, he took the opportunity to return. Accordingly, during the latter part of 1908, Cecil gave up his job with the GWR and took his family to live in Poole Keynes, where their second son, Cecil John Packer (better known as 'Jack'), was born on the 23rd August 1909. Jack's birth certificate showed that his father had indeed been successful in his change of job and was by then described as a 'shepherd'.

CHAPTER TWO

A POOLE KEYNES SHEPHERD

There is a considerable difference between the job of a farm or railway labourer and that of a shepherd, so it is interesting to ponder how Cecil was able to move into that rather specialist line of work. Jonathan Brown's book *Shepherds and Shepherding* notes that, while some shepherds followed their fathers into the job or were hired by recommendation, 'many shepherds moved into the job from other work on the farm after, perhaps, a number of years spent as a general labourer. The farm labourer drafted in to help with the sheep at busy times such as lambing, dipping and shearing, gradually gained knowledge and skill until he was able to find work as a shepherd in his own right.'

Cecil's previous farming work and connections in the village may therefore have been of some help in obtaining his new job. However and perhaps more importantly, there was also a family link with shepherding. Flo's maternal grandfather, Henry Harris, had spent all of his life as a shepherd working on many different farms across Hampshire, Wiltshire and Berkshire. He was living in the hamlet of Fosbury on the Wiltshire/Hampshire border in 1907 when his wife, Mary, died on the 23rd July. The 1911 census next shows him with Flo's parents in their cottage at 117 Poole Keynes, so it seems that Henry moved in to live with his daughter and son-in-law shortly after Mary's death. In such a circumstance Henry and Cecil must have known each other, so Henry would have been able to provide advice and encouragement to Cecil regarding his decision to seek employment as a shepherd.

No. 117 Poole Keynes was one of three cottages and various other buildings all known as 'Oakwell' and located about midway between Poole Keynes and Oaksey, close to the Gloucestershire/Wiltshire county border. No. 117 was an end cottage consisting of a single kitchen/living room downstairs, being separated from no. 116 by each cottage's wash-house. These small rooms were entered from the outside – no. 117 from the front and the other from the rear. Two bedrooms upstairs completed the accommodation. This meant that, just as with Thomas's cottage mentioned earlier, it must have been overflowing with people, because living there, or at least staying there on the night of the 1911 census (Sunday the 2nd April), were Frank and Sarah Davis, their sons Albert, Charles, Walter and Arthur, whose ages ranged from nine to 21, and 72-year-old Henry, as well as Frank's nephew, 14-year-old Joseph Harris.

Following their return to the village Cecil and Flo moved to no. 105 Poole Keynes, a cottage tied to Glebe Farm where Cecil had obtained his job. The farm, originally built in 1812 and described as a 'cottage in Poole Field' before being considerably altered, formed part of the Biddulph family's extensive estates in the area. It was occupied by the farm bailiff, who in 1901 was Frank Jennings, but by 1911 Frank had been replaced by his older brother William. The farm was located in open countryside about half a mile north of the village, and had been given various names over the years, being known as Poole Field Farm as well as Glebe Farm. The use of the term 'Glebe Farm' indicates that the farm could have been built on 'glebe' land, which is, or was, land owned by the Church. By the time of Cecil's coming back to Poole Keynes the farm was quite a sizable undertaking, being, in common with most other farms in the area, a mixed farm, and extending to some 200 acres in size. Mixed farming combined the keeping of livestock such as cattle and sheep together with arable farming; this approach was traditionally adopted to spread the risk in the event of any one crop or product failing.

Rural wages at the time amounted to something between 13 and 15 shillings per week, so Cecil was earning less than when he had worked for the GWR, although shepherds could often earn more than other farm workers and there is no reason to suppose that his wages weren't in line with those amounts. The 1905 Biddulph Estate rent book also showed the rent for Cecil's cottage to have been £2.12 shillings annually, which equates to a rent of one shilling per week. If it remained at that sort of level when Cecil moved in, it was obviously much less expensive than the house in Swindon, so it will have helped to offset any lessening of his wages.

Whatever the wages Cecil did receive, he still needed to apply for charitable relief from the Parish – just the same as his father Thomas, as well as his father-in-law Frank Davis. The parish records show that Cecil received payments of 'poor money' from 1910 until 1915 varying between 2/10d and 5/6d. Although increased social legislation by central government, such as the 1911 National Insurance Act, gradually removed the need for reliance on the Parish for assistance, the provision of parochial relief continued well into the 1920s. Frank Davis, for example, was still receiving 'poor money' as late as 1927.

Number 105 Poole Keynes formed part of a short terrace of four cottages facing the monument in the centre of the village and numbered from 102 to 105. No. 102 is thought to have been built for a farm manager, being slightly larger and constructed of dressed stone compared to the rough stone of the other cottages, which were also later in date. However, by the time of Cecil's arrival, both it and no. 103 were occupied by farm workers, while an elderly widow lived in no. 104.

The monument located immediately in front of the cottages was described by Fred Thacker as 'an old cross base upon which in 1887 a modern pillar was erected to commemorate the jubilee year of Queen Victoria's reign.' However a plaque on the side of the Cross states it to have been 'restored' in that year rather than having been freshly erected.

Cecil and Flo's new home could not have been more different from their modern house in Swindon. It was a typical old and tiny village cottage, plainly constructed of rough Cotswold stone walls under a thatched roof. There was just one room on the ground floor, a kitchen/living room with a basic stone flagged floor, and the walls and ceiling were lined with a rough plaster lath, the plaster being made up of horsehair, lime and almost anything else that could be found to bulk it out. Daylight from the windows was supplemented by lamps and candles which provided just enough light for Flo to do the family's cooking on the kitchen range in the inglenook fireplace.

This room wasn't big enough to include a staircase, so a simple wooden ladder, set in the corner, led to the single bedroom above. This was probably partitioned into two sleeping areas by a curtain hung from the cross-beam at ceiling level, although in this case there was no ceiling because the room was merely open to the underside of the thatch. Cecil's son Dennis later recalled that, although they might not always see anything, they could often hear the wildlife as it rustled among the thatch above their heads, while insects and suchlike sometimes dropped down on them. Good natural light was provided by a single window set in the gable end overlooking the yard of nearby Church Farm, while two further windows to the front were set low down close to the floor.

A small lean-to wash-house at the back of the cottage

contained the copper for boiling the water, which was drawn by bucket from a well in the garden of no. 106 Poole Keynes opposite. As with nearly every other facet of their lives, the provision of water was the polar opposite of that which had applied in Swindon. For example the town's Health Report for that year had stated: 'Practically the whole of the Borough area is supplied with water by a direct service from the Corporation mains. There are but few wells now remaining in the town, and they are being gradually closed as they are discovered to be polluted'. Yet here were Cecil and Flo relying on the provision of their water from a well in a neighbour's garden.

To supplement the supply of water from the well, rainwater was also collected and generally used for washing. Coal was stored in a corner of the wash-house for use in the range, which Flo had to clean and relight every morning. The large common rear garden area also contained a single privy which was shared with all the neighbours. When the cottages were much later altered and merged to form the pair of houses that are there now, this old toilet building was demolished and the stone from its walls recycled to build a new front porch.

Cecil's small cottage was now beginning to fill up, with two adults and two children all sharing a single bedroom, and more children would eventually join them.

Looking at the differences between their past and present lifestyles, it would be easy to conclude that they might regret their move away from Swindon. But it is much more likely that Cecil and Flo both felt that this change was a price well worth paying to see the improvement to Cecil's health brought about by his now working in the fresh air of the countryside. There was also, of course, the added advantage of living so much closer to both of their families.

However, it wasn't just Cecil and Flo's accommodation that was in striking contrast to their previous life in Swindon; everything had changed. Perhaps Poole Keynes' considerably less frantic way of life was one of the reasons that brought them back to the village. Cecil's walk to and from work, for example, couldn't have been more different from his corresponding walk to work in Swindon. Instead of making his way from Albion Street along the busy Rodbourne Road, thronged with many hundreds of other workmen, his route to work in the village was solitary and pastoral.

When he was needed at the farm he walked there through the fields rather than simply following the road because it avoided the road's dog-leg bend. Turning left out of his front door, Cecil walked as far as the road's sharp bend leading to the church and then crossed over to the right. Here he stepped over a stone stile (which is no longer there) and followed the footpath as it angled across a field to a place where the field's boundary hedge abuts the road. Passing through a gap in the hedge, his walk continued onwards to a point just north of a small group of bushes where the path joined the road. Cecil then took the path beside the road for the remaining couple of hundred yards or so before reaching the farm and its rick yard over a second stone stile, which can still be seen today.

Apart from exchanging the hustle and bustle of the railway town with its busy shopping streets for the quiet country lanes of the village, Cecil and Flo were now only served by a single tiny shop located in a stone and tile lean-to structure attached to the side of no. 106. The shop closed many years ago and was incorporated into the living accommodation of the house. However a hint of the property's previous use was revealed during a subsequent refurbishment. Quite incredibly, considerable traces of flour dust were found covered in layers of paint on the doorway connecting the former shop and house. It is also still possible to see where there was an opening in the cottage's garden wall allowing customers to gain access to the shop.

The Medlicott family had lived at no. 106 since at least 1851, and widow Elizabeth Medlicott was listed at the property as a 'Grocer' in the 1891 census, while her son George had taken over the business and was listed as a 'Haulier & Grocer' in 1901. Kelly's 1906 directory then listed him as 'Shopkeeper and Carrier departing from the Three Compasses in Cirencester every Monday and Friday' but, although the 1911 census simply listed him as a 'Farmer & Carrier,' he was still shown as 'Shopkeeper & Carrier' in the 1914 Kelly's Directory. The Carrier, of course, was a major point of contact with much of the world outside Poole Keynes, carrying both goods and passengers, albeit on a rather limited basis, between the village and Cirencester or the local railway station at Kemble.

The near total absence of any shopping facilities in the village was matched only by the complete absence of any 'places of entertainment' or even a village pub. If Cecil felt that he would like a pint of beer he would have had to go to the Bakers Arms, which was about a mile away in Somerford Keynes, or he could go a slightly further 1½ miles and visit the Wheatsheaf in Oaksey.

However the tranquillity of life in Poole Keynes could still be readily disturbed as the young men of the village, including Cecil's younger brother Rowland, sometimes engaged in activities which provoked the intervention of the law. The *Cheltenham Chronicle* newspaper for Saturday 1st October 1910 reported that

'Frank Medlicott, Henry Rouse, Rowland Packer, Harry Rigsby and Edward Hardy, young men of Poole Keynes, were summonsed for wilful damage to the extent of £3 to a steam engine and engine sheet and a barn door, the property of Mr W Large, farmer on Sept 15, which was alleged to have been done by the firing of a gun'. The *Gloucester Citizen* also reported that David Jerram, an engine driver working for Mr Large 'testified to the condition of the engine and its subsequent damage' while PC Hirons of Kemble 'produced a number of flattened bullets which had been picked up in the barn'.

It seems that these young men had clubbed together to buy a gun because, according to Edward Hardy in their defence at the hearing, 'they had read in the newspapers that their first duty was the defence of their country.' The young men had then decided to practise in the gun's use by shooting at a piece of paper attached to the door of a barn in the village. However their unfortunate lack of accuracy had resulted in damage to the engine which was kept inside the barn. Although they all denied the charge, it was reported that 'the defendants were fined 2/6d and ordered to pay 6s each towards the damage'; and as Mr Large employed Rowland's father, Thomas, it is highly likely that Rowland will have experienced a considerable degree of parental (as well as legal) chastisement for his participation in this particular incident. Cecil's reaction to his brother's appearance before the magistrates is not recorded.

This target practice may well have taken place fairly close to Lower Farm, where, in the large field across the road and to the east of the farmhouse, there was a building commonly known as the 'tractor shed'. This barn-type structure was screened from Lower Farm by another building and to the south and east by extensive and thickly-planted orchards, thereby providing a convenient and concealed location for the village lads to practise their marksmanship (or lack of it).

Cecil's new job as a shepherd filled an important role on the farm. A textbook by W Fream published in 1891 (*The Elements of Agriculture*) had described the shepherd as 'a very important person on a sheep-breeding farm; and a shepherd who understands his duties, and can perform them efficiently, is a well-qualified man of sound experience.' Edith Brill's book *Life and Tradition on the Cotswolds* notes that 'the shepherd came top in the hierarchy of farm-workers subject to no man but the farmer himself, and a farmer with a good shepherd knew better than to insist too strongly on his own way.' Additionally, according to a mid-nineteenth century farming encyclopaedia, he was 'one of the choicest of rural men.' This position in the farming community is confirmed by Edith Brill, who further wrote: 'other workers could be easily replaced, but not a shepherd. He was the only one given his rank; head carters, ploughmen, stock men were known by their names but he was 'Shep', or 'Shepherd', a title of respect'. Indeed this tradition is acknowledged locally in Poole Keynes, where Cecil was also accorded the special nickname or title of 'Shep Packer'.

According to Jonathan Brown the shepherd was in a position of great trust, having charge of the flock and often being free to organise his own work. The farmer or, in this case William Jennings, the farm bailiff, had almost no influence over him, and even had to defer to him at times. Persuading the shepherd to leave his fields to help out at harvest time, for example, could require the utmost diplomacy on the part of the farmer or bailiff. We shall never really know if Cecil was like this as a shepherd, but I would like to think that he was sufficiently well regarded and good at his job to be able, in the words of Wiltshire author A G Street, to 'condescend to come for an hour or two, as one conferring a favour'.

Cecil's life as a shepherd was punctuated by a series of regular events through the year. The cycle began in the autumn when the ram was put to the ewe in a procedure known as 'tupping'. This was followed by lambing, and weaning of lambs, in the spring and then by shearing and dipping in the early summer.

The time to start the tupping could vary with the need for lambing. The ewe's gestation period is exactly 21 weeks, so tupping could be arranged for the birth of the lambs to occur whenever they were needed. The availability of spring grass to feed the ewes and lambs was originally used to determine the calculation of the time, but when Cecil was a shepherd, the greater use of turnips and feed gave him increased flexibility in arranging matters, although his work could never be entirely independent of the seasons. Whatever the timing, the tupping was generally spread over a period of 3-4 weeks, to give a similar spread of births in the lambing season. Having spent his time so far in relative idleness, the ram had to be brought into condition before he was introduced to the ewes, so Cecil had to give him some exercise, even to the extent of taking him for walks, rather as one would walk a dog.

Before the lambs were due, Cecil built small lambing pens of wattle for them. These were formed from moveable hurdles made of interwoven willow or hazel sticks, which provided an enclosed space where the ewes could have their lambs. Alan Stanford, whose house now incorporates no. 117 where Flo's parents lived, recalled that the area behind their garden was originally very damp and waterlogged, and said it 'was covered in willows'. This is clearly indicated on the 1900 OS map, so I think it most likely that this is where Cecil obtained the wood he used to construct the pens. There was also a plentiful supply of hazel trees along the adjacent hedge lines which could also have provided wood to make the hurdles. Cecil could well have learnt his hurdle-making skills from Henry Harris before taking the cut sticks up to Glebe Farm to construct the pens in the farm's rick yard. This was situated on the opposite side of the road just south of the farmhouse, and was a courtyard type arrangement with a large and traditional stone-built barn together with cow sheds, pigsties and stabling to one side. The yard and buildings were all linked by a strong stone wall, thereby ensuring that the ewes and lambs, in the words of Ronnie Roe, would be 'safe from the foxes and stuff'. Ronnie remembered 'about eleven ricks in there: a row of corn ricks – beautiful up on staddle stones you know – and then the lambing pens were all around the outside'. Staddle stones are mushroom-shaped stones which support a rick, keeping it off the ground and so preventing rodents from getting inside. The stones are now in the garden of the farmhouse.

Lambing was just about the most crucial time of year for Cecil because so much depended on it being successful, as it formed a major part of the farm's income. According to Ronnie Roe, a shepherd such as Cecil would have had to be 'on duty, day and night. He had his hut in the yard with a little chimney going – his stove – and he was on hand to look after any weakly lambs or that, right through the night'. Looking after these new-born lambs in particular was a task ideally suited to Cecil's caring disposition. W.J. Malden, in a textbook written before 1914, advised: 'the shepherd shall not be given any other work to do during the busiest season of lambing' because the ewes and lambs needed constant attention, for example in ensuring that mothers were accepting their lambs. Cecil also had to keep a watchful eye on these new lambs during their first few weeks to ensure that they settled in the fields before he docked their tails, usually after about 12 weeks, as a precaution against disease.

One interesting, and somewhat unconventional, treatment for the care of newly-born lambs that I came across in my researches is described in Elspeth Huxley's fascinating book *Gallipot Eyes*. Referring to life in nearby Oaksey, she writes of an old shepherd who was 'knowledgeable about the needs of lambs' and who told her: 'if a lamb's dropped cold and wet, warm milk will curdle in its stomach. Give it a drop of gin, now, no more than a teaspoon, and the milk won't curdle'. This shepherd apparently always carried a bottle of gin in his pocket and recorded that he 'never lost a lamb.' I think it is quite possible that giving a teaspoon of gin to a needy new-born lamb was a procedure that Cecil may well have heard about and possibly even relied upon.

Ronnie explained that the farm's large flock of sheep consisted of the big Oxford Down breed. These sheep have brown/black faces, weigh anything between 250-300lb and produce the heaviest fleeces of any of the Down breeds. When helping with the lambing and going to check on the condition of the lambs in the pens, Ronnie talked of what 'fearful creatures' they could be. 'They'd come at you and they would stamp,' he said. He remembered the shepherd telling him to go and look in the pens, saying: 'It's all right. She won't hurt you. You go and tell me how many lambs there are in there.' He described the weaning pens as 'lovely and warm and comfortable. There were one or two or sometimes three lambs in behind there'.

It was during this lambing season that the 'shepherd's hut,' the use of which dates back to the 15th Century, will have truly proved its value to Cecil. The 'hut' was basically a portable caravan where he could live while he cared for the ewes and their newly-born lambs. Flo was able to help during this very busy time by bringing Cecil's meals out to him, particularly while he was staying in his hut and not always able to get home. Mrs Irene Harrison of Oakwell recalled that the shepherd's huts had four wheels on them so they could be moved by horses to where they were needed. Edith Brill records that inside the hut was 'a squat iron stove with a tin pipe through the roof and a heavy pointed bar of iron for making holes in the ground for erecting hurdles.' There was also a table, a bed and space for Cecil to store his tools and 'first aid remedies for his flock'. Most huts were made wholly of wood, but during the early years of the 20th century, many were built by Messrs Reeves, of Bratton in Wiltshire, using sheets of corrugated iron on a wooden frame. These old workaday huts are now very valuable collectors' items.

Ronnie described Glebe Farm as being 'essentially sheep, roots and corn', the 'roots' consisting of mangolds, swede and turnips to feed the animals. Jonathon Brown wrote: 'rather than lift the roots, it was common to bring sheep into the fields between autumn and spring to eat the crops in situ, a system known as 'folding'.' Other crops were grown for the same purpose, including carrots, cabbage and kale. Cecil had to ensure that the sheep progressed across the field in an orderly fashion, leaving an even distribution of manure for the following crop of cereals by setting up folds within the fields.

These folds were marked off by temporary fences or

hurdles, very much like the lambing pens, and similarly constructed, with legs to hold them in place in the field. Sometimes Cecil might have needed to construct heavier wooden hurdles known as 'gate hurdles', which were like a farm gate but not quite so big. These were the heaviest of the hurdles, and he may have needed to call on one of the other farm workers to help in setting them up. The hurdles were also used for other temporary purposes such as providing protection for the ewes and their young lambs, or as stockades to corral the sheep before dipping.

There were also the farm's pasture fields, to which Cecil had to carry supplies of additional food such as oilcake, corn and chopped roots, although unlike the situation on other farms, he was fortunate in not having to make provision for the sheep to be supplied with water. While shepherds elsewhere needed to maintain separate troughs of drinking water, Cecil's sheep were able to rely on naturally-occurring ponds in the fields which were full of spring water, allowing the sheep to slake their thirst. Teresa Smith, who farms in the village, said that several of the springs were stone lined.

Poole Keynes, along with Poulton near Cirencester, is almost unique in being the location of such a high water-table which supplied these ponds – and gave the village the first word of its name - although the ponds have all largely disappeared over time, principally as a result of extensive gravel extraction in the area. Notwithstanding the assertion by HW John Cuss in his book *The Valley of the Upper Thames* that there is 'some age-old affinity' with the name of the Poole family, the name of the village actually predates them by some 500 years. 'Pole' appears in the Domesday Book as being originally a Saxon village, whereas the Pooles didn't lease 'Pole' until early in the 16th Century, so the village can't have been named after them.

As well as managing the sheep in the folds and in the field, Cecil was responsible for maintaining the quality of the flock, keeping their feet clean and sound and their bodies clean, and ensuring that they reached peak condition in time for market, and he had to do all of this as well as attending to their basic veterinary care. This could be onerous work, because sheep are prone to a variety of ailments which Cecil had to deal with largely by himself using the limited preparations available at the time, such as disinfectant and carbolic soap. Dressings, medicines, surgical tools and a metal pail for washing hands were also part of his equipment. The liquid medicines Cecil had to administer were known as 'drenches', and the cup he used to pour the medicine down the sheep's throat was a known as a 'drenching horn'. Another important item in Cecil's toolkit was his shepherds' knife, which he used for jobs such as trimming hoofs and horns and cutting string.

One common disease in sheep was 'scab', caused by parasitic ticks and lice. By the 1830s the vet William Cooper had begun to sell a mixture of arsenic and sulphur as a treatment for scab which could be applied in dilute form. It soon became apparent that the best method of applying this mixture was for the sheep to be dipped in it, and the business that Mr Cooper founded went on to become one of the country's biggest manufacturers of sheep dip.

The dipping of sheep soon became common practice, and it was made compulsory in 1907 when a policeman had to be in attendance to verify that the whole flock had been dipped correctly. Cecil, or the farm bailiff, therefore had to call upon the local policeman from Kemble to oversee the dipping process, which was carried out in the rick yard. This was not an easy task, because the sheep did not like getting wet. Accordingly plenty of men were needed to chase the recalcitrant sheep and ensure that they were completely submerged as they went through the bath along with the sheep dogs. Long-handled dipping hooks were used to push the animals under, although Cecil and the other farmworkers were still in danger of being splashed by the noxious mixture, which Irene Harrison described as having a 'revolting smell.' The requirement for compulsory dipping was eventually brought to an end in 1991.

Obviously another important job was shearing, which generally lasted from June to early July, and which for Cecil was a very busy time. The first task in the shearing procedure was to wash the sheep to rid the fleece of any accumulated grease. This wasn't always strictly necessary, but wool that had been washed generally attracted a higher price than unwashed wool, so Cecil had to organise this work. The washing place most often used for the Glebe Farm sheep was a deep pool at the edge of Kemble village and approached from Poole Keynes along the appropriately named 'Washpool Lane' to the north of Glebe Farm. The site still exists but is now considerably overgrown, and the tree growth makes it difficult to imagine that there was ever a sheep 'washing pool' at that place. Additionally this site, just like the ponds in the fields, has been seriously affected by gravel extraction, so that it is now many years since any depth of water has been seen there. Sometimes, if the sheep needed to be washed in running water, Cecil drove them further on, to one of the various washing places found in the infant River Thames.

Cecil then had to call on the other farmworkers for their help in rounding up the sheep and bringing them to the wash, because the sheep disliked the washing just as much as they did the dipping. This resulted in much jostling as the animals tried to avoid getting wet which, in turn, could end up with the men being dragged into the water and getting soaked themselves. Gordon Ayres of Kemble described these big sheep to me as being 'very difficult for the men to handle'. The practice of washing the sheep on the farm died out during the 1960s, when it was replaced by the use of more effective washing machines in the wool-processing factories.

Having potentially suffered the pain and indignity of being knocked over and trampled by the sheep during the washing process, Cecil next had to undertake the actual job of shearing the sheep. This was a difficult task which involved holding the sheep with one hand while using the other to shear the animal using a specially designed one-handed shearing tool with a triangular blade. Jonathan Brown wrote in his book that the task of shearing sheep was 'a skill requiring stamina to hold down sheep that would prefer to be elsewhere' while Irene Harrison described it as 'a dangerous job because the sheep often kicked out when being sheared' – and, of course, Cecil was working with very big and very heavy sheep. Once the sheep had been sheared they were marked and tallied, while Gordon Ayres said that the shorn fleeces were then rolled up and put into wool sacks before being weighed and sent by cart to the market in Cirencester for sale.

Although Cirencester's traditional wool market had declined considerably by the beginning of the 20th century, annual wool sales conducted by local auctioneer Mr A F Hobbs were still a regular occurrence in the town. Newspaper advertisements and reports of the time indicate that the sales were held at the Brewery Maltings in Cricklade Street and were often attended by 'buyers from the North of England, Scotland and the chief buying centres'. The *Cheltenham Chronicle* of 28th June 1913 for example reported that the most recent sale had seen wool from Southdown sheep make 'the best prices', fetching between 1s 3d and 1s 3½d per lb, while wool from unwashed fleeces only sold for 9½d to 11¼d.

When the 1911 Census was taken on the night of Sunday 2nd April to Monday 3rd April, Cecil, Flo, Frank and John were all still living at 105 Poole Keynes, and Cecil was continuing in his job as a 'Shepherd on Farm.' Later that year on the 18th August a third son, Dennis Edward, was born; the Birth Certificate confirmed the family's address as 105 Poole Keynes and that Cecil was still working as a shepherd.

The birth of fourth son Leslie Kenneth Packer, on the 4th January 1914, heralded the start of a momentous year. The assassination of an obscure member of the Austro-Hungarian royal family in faraway Sarajevo on the 28th June seems to have had little or no impact in the quiet village where Cecil continued to work peaceably at his job. Indeed I couldn't find any reference at all to the event in the local newspapers, which, even as the international political situation deteriorated, were far more concerned with matters closer to home. In retrospect, it seems astonishing to me that so many people were apparently blissfully unaware of the catastrophe which was about to engulf them. However, the local situation was perhaps simply representative of a much wider failure to appreciate what was about to happen, probably best described by Winston Churchill in a letter to his wife on the 28th July when he wrote of Europe being in a 'kind of dull cataleptic trance'.

Amongst the sundry adverts for the likes of a two-seater Ford car for £125, Black Cat Cigarettes at 2½d and 3d and Lux Washing Powder – 'Pour Lux on the troubled waters of the wash' (costing between 1d and 4d) – were more humdrum news items: Cirencester Police Court fined a man seven shillings for using 'bad language' in Watermoor Road, a student from the Royal Agricultural College was fined a similar seven shillings for 'riding a bicycle to the danger of the public,' and the Earl of Suffolk & Berkshire was reported to have returned to town from Paris. One major topic of conversation in Poole Keynes that summer was a terrific hailstorm in July which, according to Ronnie Roe, 'lashed the whole village causing extensive damage: broke windows and all sorts'.

The arrival of the storm, however, could well have been predicted by the Poole Keynes 'weather gauge' – the Swindon to Gloucester railway line. This passes through open countryside about half a mile to the west of the village, but the passage of the trains is rarely heard in the village itself unless, that is, the wind is blowing from that direction. Under those circumstances the sound of the trains can clearly be heard, being carried along by the westerly wind and heralding the arrival of rain. This has led to the village's weather-forecasting rhyme, with which I am sure Cecil must have been familiar: 'If you can hear the train, then it's going to rain'. I can also vouch for the accuracy of this forecasting method, having experienced it myself. I was walking along the road from Glebe Farm to the village one sunny afternoon in July 2015 when for the first time I heard the roar of a passing train and learned then of the rhyme. Within a matter of hours the warm weather disappeared, to be followed by heavy rain and driving winds.

National news concentrated on the principle issues at the time, such as the question of Irish Home Rule and the campaigns of the suffragette movement, while subordinate reports covered such subjects as agitation over agricultural wages (although that issue appears to have largely bypassed Poole Keynes), the delayed Budget, and the Bill to formally abandon the Wilts and Berks Canal. In fact it wasn't until the 31st July that the first reference to 'the crisis' appeared in the papers, but even then, it was a crisis that only seemed to concern others. One newspaper printed a helpful article listing the 'principle armies which might be involved in hostilities arising out of the current crisis.' The list included 'Austria-Hungary, Servia, Russia, Germany, France and Italy', but wholly omitted England, which was cast in the role of concerned bystander. Indeed this was a view shared by senior politicians; Prime Minister Herbert Asquith wrote, in reference to the growing crisis, that he saw 'no reason why we should be anything more than spectators'. Other newspaper headlines referred to Austria's declaration of war and the 'Grave Outlook', but even that level of interest was eclipsed by numerous reports concerning the usual local round of summer garden fetes, bazaars and flower shows.

However everything changed on the 4th August 1914 when Britain declared war on Germany, and a flurry of

'War Stories' now spilled across the pages of the papers. One of the Government's first moves thereafter was to appoint Field Marshal the Earl Kitchener of Khartoum as Secretary of State for War on the 6th August. Kitchener was fully aware that the regular British Army was too small for extended campaigning on the European mainland and, importantly, had also concluded that the war would not be over by Christmas as was thought by many at the time. Accordingly he made plans to increase the size of the Army from six to seventy Divisions and to plan for a war that would last at least three years.

There then followed a massive poster and newspaper crusade appealing for the first hundred thousand men to volunteer for the 'New Army', or the 'Kitchener Army', as it became known. This appeal was directed at all men aged between 19 and 30 who were asked to join up for three years or the duration of the war, whichever was the longer. During August alone nearly 300,000 men responded to the call for volunteers, while nearly three million had joined by the end of the year, and another million and a quarter in 1915. This represented the considerable figure of just under one in eleven of the total population of Great Britain and Ireland – and somewhere amongst this mighty flood of volunteers was 29-year-old father of four Cecil Thomas Packer.

So what was it that caused Cecil to join up? Many young men at the time joined up seeking adventure, but he had already taken that route when he was 18 and found that army life was not for him. Additionally he was no longer that young – he now had a growing family, an important job and responsibilities. Alternatively, and possibly more likely, he could have joined up out of a sense of patriotism, as so very many did during a time when people had an enormous and deeply-felt sense of pride in their country. However his decision could equally have been prompted by the recent death in action of his brother-in-law, 22-year-old Francis John Davis. John, as he was commonly known, was a regular soldier and by 1911 he was serving with the 1st Battalion of the Gloucestershire Regiment based at Cambridge Barracks in Portsmouth. However by the outbreak of war in 1914 he was stationed at Tientsin in China with the Glosters 2nd Battalion, which soon received orders to join the British Expeditionary Force in France.

They landed at Le Havre on the 18th December and moved to take up positions on the front line around the medieval town of Ypres in Belgium. The town occupied a key position on the route leading to the French coastal ports of Calais and Dunkirk, and it was therefore regarded as important to both the British and the

Germans; the British, in particular, were determined to defend it at all costs. The 1st Battle of Ypres, which is often said to have seen the death of the pre-war professional army, ended in November, but fighting had continued intermittently since then as the opposing armies probed each other's positions, and the dark winter days of 1914/1915 were marked by the thunder of artillery barrages interspersed by the crack of rifle fire as snipers picked off the unwary.

Private Edgar Corble of the Rifle Brigade was stationed in the same general area of the front line as was John Davis and his story, published in the *Old Masonians' Gazette,* contained this description of life in that locality: 'The relatively calm period between 3rd November and the 2nd battle of Ypres on 22nd April was one of great discomfort; a period in which men grew old in a single night, so terrible were the conditions of life in the trenches during the first winter of the war. Trench warfare was in its infancy, sandbags were scarce.' The often still too shallow trenches provided scant protection against snipers. The trenches were 'absolute quagmires, water and mud ankle deep, knee deep in slime, the stench of the unburied dead'. Nonetheless the soldiers '...settled down quickly to their new life and cheerfully improvised to make themselves as comfortable as possible. Letters, food parcels and comforts from home eased the awfulness of the first wet, cold winter in the crude early trenches.'

John's battalion was occupying trenches around the village of Dickebusch, some three miles or so to the south-west of Ypres, when he was killed on the 18th January 1915. The sandbag scarcity described above seems to have left him poorly protected, which led to him falling victim to a German sniper. I think his death was a graphic illustration of the point made by Mark Adkin that 'the fighting on the Western Front never stopped... there were quiet periods and quieter parts of the front but men were fighting and dying somewhere every hour of every day of the 52 months that the war lasted'.

A report of John's death subsequently appeared on the 30th January in the *Wilts & Gloucestershire Standard,* which printed the letter from Lt L Lachlan, John's Platoon Commander, to his parents containing the heart-breaking news. Lt Lachlan wrote that John 'was shot at about 1.30pm yesterday 18 Jan, in the trenches. I am thankful to say that death was almost instantaneous, and that he had no pain. I am pleased to be able to let you know that he has been buried with all decency and a small wooden cross has been erected over his grave. He was a good fellow and did good work, and I am awfully sorry to lose him.'

Sadly it seems that John's grave was lost in the heavy fighting which subsequently engulfed the area, and he now has no known grave, although he is commemorated on the Menin Gate Memorial at Ypres. Cecil enlisted very shortly after receiving the news of John's death, so perhaps his decision to join the Army flowed from a sense of responsibility and a desire to 'finish the job' that his brother-in-law had started in order that John's death should not have been in vain.

CHAPTER THREE

SENT TO GALLIPOLI

Based on his Army number of 20550, it seems that Cecil, for whatever motive, answered Kitchener's call and joined up in April 1915. He enlisted in the Gloucestershire Regiment at Cirencester and was sent to join the 7th (Service) Battalion of the Regiment, which had been formed in Bristol during August 1914. The term 'Service Battalion' was applied to all of Kitchener's 'New Army' units and was indicative of the fact that the men in the battalion were effectively recruited to serve only for the duration of the war. The title also showed that the men in these units were recruited for 'General Service' as opposed to 'Home

Service' and helped to distinguish them from Regular, Reserve and Territorial Force units.

Despite the passing of 11 years since his first encounter with the place, Cecil must surely have experienced some feeling of trepidation as he arrived once more at the Gloucestershire Regiment's Horfield Depot for his initial training. However he was now there under entirely different circumstances. On this occasion he was preparing to fight for his country in time of war and peril and to continue the work of his late brother-in-law, rather than to simply engage in the apparent adventures of peace-time soldiering.

Cecil's training at the depot included spending some six and a half hours each day practising marching drill and learning to handle the standard issue British Army rifle. This was the bolt action .303in Short Magazine Lee Enfield (SMLE), which first came into service in 1895 and would remain in service until 1957. The rifle weighed 8.8lb and was 44" long with a maximum range of some 2,000 yards, although its effective range was around 550 yards. The magazine held 10 bullets in a clip of two five-round charges which could be quickly loaded by placing them in the magazine and pushing down with the thumb. Described as 'a robust and reliable weapon', the rifle could be used with a 21" sword bayonet clipped on the end. I can remember being

taught how to use this weapon during my time in the
Army Cadet Force at school in the late 1960s; it had a
ferocious kick when being fired so you had to hold the
gun very tightly against your shoulder or it could
seriously damage your collar bone.

The training period in Bristol lasted for around two
months before Cecil and the other recruits were sent to
Purfleet in Essex, where the 'feeder battalion' for the
Front Line practised its firing. Here recruits were firstly
engaged in simply marking the firing for more advanced
soldiers before eventually being allowed to do their own
shooting. After about a month or so of this firing
training, Cecil was probably sent on some brief home
leave before his departure to join the main body of the
battalion.

The 7th (Service) Battalion had been allocated upon
its formation to the 39th Brigade of the British Army's
13th (Western) Division. The division had assembled at
Tidworth on the edge of Salisbury Plain in late August
1914 and then gone into billets at Basingstoke in
January 1915. At the end of February 1915 it was
concentrated at Blackdown near Aldershot in
Hampshire, and then, on the 19th June 1915, it sailed
from Avonmouth for the Gallipoli Peninsula, landing
there on the 11th July.

The Dardanelles, or Gallipoli, Campaign was an

attempt by British, Dominion and French forces to capture Turkey's Dardanelles Strait, which connects the Black Sea with the Mediterranean. The aim was to knock Turkey out of the war and to relieve pressure on the Russians. An Anglo-French fleet had tried to force the Strait in February 1915, but this had not been successful, so troops in support of the enterprise had been landed on the Gallipoli Peninsula in April. These had incurred heavy losses for no significant gains, so reinforcements were despatched in support, thereby resulting in what writer and former Army officer Richard Awdry described as 'one of the greatest disasters of the War'.

The 7th Battalion had been heavily involved in the furious Gallipoli battles, including that of the 6th August, when every officer and senior NCO in the battalion had either been killed or wounded, although the men had continued fighting heroically. The battalion was therefore in desperate need of the draft of reinforcements, including Cecil, that left England on the 28th August together with some 2,000 other troops, who all embarked at Southampton on board His Majesty's Troopship *Mauretania*. This was a fast transatlantic liner launched in 1906, and sister ship to the ill-fated *Lusitania*, which had been sunk off Ireland by a German U Boat earlier in the year.

Cecil's Medal Card indicates that he arrived in the 'Dardanelles Theatre of War' on the 23rd September 1915. This was probably at the Army's main reception area near Mudros, a small Greek port on the Aegean island of Lemnos which provided a convenient base for gathering troops destined for Gallipoli. Alan Moorehead's book *Gallipoli* describes the depressing sight of the camp: 'Mudros, like every transit camp in every war, was awful: a city of dusty tents, the dreary anonymous hutments on the wharves, the appalling canteen food eaten amongst strangers'. After a brief spell there while all the various reinforcements were assembled, Cecil was next landed on the Gallipoli peninsula itself.

The dreadful summer fighting had finished by the time Cecil reached the war zone, the various British advances having been defeated by poor generalship and dogged Turkish resistance, although the Turks were not strong enough to force the British back. Therefore, and just as was the case on the Western Front in France, the two sides were stalemated and simply hanging on awaiting developments. These were not slow in coming, because, on 25th September and coinciding with Cecil's arrival, two Army divisions (one British and one French) were removed from the battle-line on the orders of the Government and despatched for service in Salonica (now Thessalonica) in Greece. The Commander-In-Chief of the Dardanelles forces, Sir Ian Hamilton, could now see that political support for the Gallipoli Campaign was fast dwindling and that this first reduction in troop numbers could well signal the beginning of the campaign's end.

The War Diary for the 39th Infantry Brigade on the 27th September records that 'During the night a draft for the Glosters of one Officer and 90 Other Ranks arrived and was taken up to the trenches.' The 'night' referred to in the War Diary entry was probably the night of 26th/27th September because the 7th Battalion's War Diary for 26th September states 'Lieut Miller and draft of 95 men arrived'. Although the numbers of soldiers recorded in the two diaries are different, this was almost certainly the same draft referred to in the brigade's War Diary. Reinforcements were nearly always brought up to the front-line trenches under the cover of darkness at night to minimise casualties from sniper fire amongst those inexperienced in the very great dangers inherent in trench warfare. It is almost certain that Cecil was amongst this freshly-arrived group of soldiers.

An Army battalion was generally regarded as the soldier's 'home' and, at full strength, could total something around a thousand men under the command of a Lieutenant Colonel. However, when Cecil arrived on the peninsula, the effective strength of his battalion was recorded in its War Diary on the 25th September as being a mere 533 men. This figure illustrates the horrifying impact of the fighting during the summer and the urgent need for the battalion to be reinforced by men such as Cecil and his comrades. The battalion was usually made up of four companies, each under the command of a Major or Captain, with the company being divided into four platoons of around 40 men each commanded by a Subaltern (a Lieutenant or 2nd Lieutenant). It was the platoon which essentially formed Cecil's army 'family'; in describing the life of a private soldier, Mark Adkins wrote, 'it was with these close comrades that he ate, slept, worked and fought.' The platoon was then sub-divided into four sections, each of which was under the charge of a Corporal.

The battalion's War Diary also records that the battalion was then occupying trenches near Sulijik Farm in the Anafarta Valley, which is located on the northernmost Suvla section of the landings where the beaches are linked to a large inland dry salt lake. The Australian and New Zealand troops were to the south at the Anzac beachhead, while more British troops were on the bottom tip of the peninsula at Cape Helles.

Once he had arrived in the trenches, Cecil's first

experience of trench warfare came quite quickly. The diary entry for 27th September records that 'at 7.15pm heavy firing broke out on our right' and this was followed by firing from both sides all along the line. During this time some 6,000 rounds of ammunition were discharged, with one man being killed and six wounded. The diary records little activity for the remainder of the month except that three more men lost their lives – all presumably killed by sniper fire.

The 3rd October saw the battalion's strength recorded as being 8 Officers and 3 attached plus 550 Other Ranks when it was relieved by the North Staffordshire Regiment and moved to the reserve trenches. Although not mentioned in the diary, a foretaste of the difficult winter weather ahead occurred on the 8th October when a gale blew up. The heavy seas caused some of the provisioning barges at Suvla Bay to break loose and destroy a large section of the pier. Then just a few days later, on the 11th October, Lord Kitchener sent a cable to General Hamilton asking for an estimate of the number of casualties likely to be caused in the event that the Peninsula was to be evacuated. This was a further sign that political support at home for the campaign was fast ebbing away. Hamilton's estimate of 50% casualties caused the Government serious concern but was then rejected as being too alarmist.

Hamilton was also the subject of serious personal criticism in London and was accordingly replaced on the 15th October by General Sir Charles Monroe. The General was described in Volume 6 of the war's Standard History as being 'a General who had greatly distinguished himself in the campaigns in France and Flanders'. Winston Churchill however delivered a more withering assessment of the General, writing that he 'was an officer of quick decision. He came, he saw, he capitulated.'

Meanwhile, in the trenches, the Glosters' period in reserve lasted until the 24th October. It was by no means free of danger to Cecil and his comrades because during that supposedly quieter period alone, three men were killed and 12 wounded. Reinforcements continued to arrive on a regular basis, and the battalion's strength on 22nd October is shown as 22 Officers and 671 men. However these arrivals were rarely sufficient to offset the daily wastage from sickness, particularly amongst the longer-serving soldiers. The battalion's return to the trenches, when they reoccupied their old positions held by the North Staffordshire Regiment, coincided with the arrival of a further draft of 50 reinforcements from Mudros. However the battalion continued to suffer a steady and relentless drain of casualties – two men killed and two wounded on the 26th October, four men wounded on the 27th October and one on the 28th October, at which point the battalion's strength is recorded as 22 Officers + 3 attached and 676 men.

The 29th October saw two men wounded and a note in the War Diary to the effect that 'Turk patrols rather active in front.' A further two men were wounded on the 30th October, the day General Monroe made a tour of the positions on the peninsula and discussed the situation with his Divisional and Corps Commanders. As the month drew to a close, 50 more men arrived to reinforce the battalion from England while General Monroe made his formal recommendation to the British Government that the army should be evacuated.

November started as October had ended, with a daily drain of casualties, although the causes are not always specified in the diary. Lord Kitchener also arrived in Gallipoli at this time and undertook a three-day tour of the positions, much in the fashion of General Monroe a short time previously. On the 15th November Kitchener reported to London, confirming General Monroe's view that evacuation of the troops was the only option available.

The weather now turned, as if confirming the need for everyone to get away from the peninsula as quickly as possible, and the Great Storm of 26th November bore down on all participants. Its immediate impact is described in the battalion's War Diary: 'At about 1830, 26/27th a rain storm coming with great rapidity and violence burst over our lines. As a result the ground between our firing line and that of the enemy quickly became the bed of a large lake, the weight and volume of which proved too great for our parapets and the water pouring in soon rendered our trenches untenable'. Cecil and the other soldiers occupying the trenches at the time had to dig themselves in behind the parados, a bank of earth and sandbags at the rear of the trench. The diary went on to record the difficulty of maintaining contact with other units on either side of the battalion and concluded with the note that 'The Flood destroyed much property equipment etc and carried away or destroyed most of the Battalion and Company records.'

However this record is either an example of typical British understatement or the battalion actually fared less badly than others. I suspect it to be the former, because the storm's impact was considerable and was best described by Alan Moorehead: 'No one... could have anticipated the horror and severity of the blizzard that swept down on the Dardanelles on November 27th 1915. Nothing like it had been known there for forty years. For the first twenty-four hours rain poured down and violent thunderstorms raged over the peninsula. Then, as the wind veered round to the north and rose to hurricane force, there followed two days of snow and icy sleet. After this there were two nights of frost.'

Moorehead went on: 'At Anzac and Cape Helles the soldiers were well dug in, and there was some small protection from the surrounding hills, but at Suvla the men were defenceless.' (Suvla was where Cecil was stationed with the 7th Battalion.) 'The earth there was so stony that in place of trenches stone parapets had been built above ground. These burst open in the first deluge, and a torrent came rushing down to the salt lake, carrying with it the bodies of the Turks who had been drowned in the hills. Soon the lake was four feet deep, and on both sides the war was forgotten. Turks and British alike jumped up on what was left of the parapets in full view of one another and there they perched, numb and shivering, while the flood went by. Then, overnight, when the landscape turned to a universal white, dysentery vanished along with the flies and dust, but the cold was past all bearing... The freeze that followed was worse than any shelling. Triggers were jammed and rifles refused to fire... Blankets and bedding were so congealed with cold they could be stood on end. Everywhere mud had turned to ice and the roofs of the dugouts were lined with icicles as hard as iron. A tacit truce prevailed along the front while the men gave themselves up to the simple struggle of finding enough warmth to remain alive. Nevinson, the war correspondent, describes how he saw men staggering down to the beaches from the trenches: 'They could neither hear nor speak, but stared about them like bewildered bullocks.'

Moorehead concluded his account, writing: 'On November 30, when the wind had blown itself out at last, a reckoning was made, and it was found that the allied army had lost one tenth of its strength. Two hundred soldiers had been drowned, 5,000 were suffering from frostbite, and another 5,000 were casualties of one sort or another.' The anonymous writer of the battalion's War Diary for this period continued with a more prosaic approach, confining himself to reports of trench rebuilding and repositioning following the destruction of the floods. Also recorded in the diary is the fact that six men were killed and 15 wounded by enemy shelling, and that three men died of exposure.

Losses in Cecil's battalion were not solely confined to his immediate friends and comrades. They were also being suffered amongst its officers, with five being admitted to hospital, although the reasons are not specified. This resulted in the somewhat odd incident on the 30th November of a Staff Captain taking command of the battalion and then being almost immediately relieved of that command by a Captain from the 6th East

Lancashire Regiment acting on the specific orders of the Divisional Commander. One can only assume that the luckless Staff Captain, seeing the battalion virtually bereft of officers, thought he had an opportunity to escape from his staff job and secure a field command, only to be then promptly hauled back by his superiors.

During the first part of December the battalion continued to suffer a steady toll of killed and wounded, although the numbers were much offset by the arrival of reinforcements, so that its effective strength by the 12th December was 15 Officers and 447 Other Ranks. In the meantime however, Dardanelles HQ had received notice of the Government's decision to order a partial evacuation of the peninsula. The Suvla and Anzac beachheads were to be abandoned but Helles was to be retained; and so the battalion's War Diary also records on the 12th December that 'preparations commenced for general evacuation, all weak men evacuated, kits and stores removed by night.'

The plan for the evacuation of the beachheads was for the bulk of the Army to make a gradual and secret withdrawal, leaving behind a rearguard of the 'bravest and the steadiest men' before they too were evacuated. The great hope was that this vast exercise would be accomplished without the knowledge of the Turks.

The contribution of Cecil's battalion to the rearguard

consisted of two Officers and 48 Other Ranks, who remained in the trenches on 17th December while their comrades moved to (A) West Beach, although there is no way of knowing to which of the particular groups Cecil belonged. The War Diary describes the battalion as having 'marched out from Sulajik,' but given the vital need for secrecy this was unlikely to have been a parade-ground affair. Upon arrival at the beach, the battalion were embarked at 17.30hrs, arriving at Mudros the following day. They then went into quarters at Mudros West Camp, where the War Diary for the 21st December recorded the battalion's effective strength as being 13 Officers and 396 Other Ranks. They were then joined by the rearguard, who arrived on the 24th December.

The stay on Mudros however was destined to be very short because, after an uneventful Christmas Day, the battalion received orders on Boxing Day that they were being sent to the Helles beachhead. Embarking on 27th December the battalion arrived on 'V' Beach at 18.30hrs before moving up to occupy positions in Gully Ravine. Nonetheless, despite the earlier decision to hold on at Cape Helles, it soon became obvious that such a situation was not possible. Large numbers of Turkish troops, relieved from containing the beachheads at Suvla and Anzac, were being moved south to reinforce their compatriots at Helles, and they would soon be sufficiently strong to strike and destroy the rather precarious Allied positions.

The Army's inability to hold on to the beachhead at Helles had at least been foreseen by one man. The Standard History quotes an anonymous British officer who presciently wrote in November 1915 that: 'Gallipoli is terrible. It is like a narrow ledge on which two men are fighting. There is no place to retreat to. The side that weakens first goes over the edge into the sea. Neither side can withdraw troops, for that would mean that one side at last would have more men than the other, and the stronger would sweep the weaker to destruction in the ocean.' Accordingly, to avoid the prediction of being swept to destruction in the ocean, the decision to evacuate Cape Helles was reached on the 28th December.

On that same day half of the battalion relieved the 4th Battalion East Lancashire Regiment at Fusiliers Bluff, while the Battalion HQ moved to Border Ravine. These manoeuvres were followed on the 29th December by the other half of the battalion moving to the Fusiliers Bluff support trenches. This repositioning was met on 30th December by sporadic Turkish artillery fire resulting in three men being killed and eight wounded. The year closed with a further two men being wounded, although the causes of these wounds are not recorded. British army infantry battalions are usually commanded by a Lieutenant Colonel, so it is indicative of the scale of losses suffered by Cecil's battalion that the War Diary for the 31st December 1915 records the battalion as being commanded by a Captain.

New Year's Day 1916 saw little activity of note except that the men in the firing line and support trenches were reinforced by a detachment of one Officer and 60 Other Ranks from the 7th North Staffs Battalion. The bulk of the battalion were moved to 'Y' Ravine in reserve on 4th January, suffering one man killed and three wounded. The Battalion's Grenadiers and Machine Gunners, however, remained in the firing line and support trenches, while the next two days then saw the battalion engaged in 'active preparations for evacuation'.

On the 7th January the diary reported: 'A Heavy Bombardment by the Turks was experienced commencing at 10.30 and lasting till 16.30 followed by Shrapnel and Machine Gun fire.' This bombardment presaged a fierce attack on the partly-evacuated lines which was bravely beaten back by the 7th North Staffs while the Glosters moved into the Support Trenches, where six men were wounded, two fatally. The battalion then spent most of the night in repairing the communication trenches and the mule track, which had been damaged in the bombardment.

In a slight change of terminology, the diary for the 8th January recorded: 'A lively Bombardment by the enemy was experienced the Turks using a great quantity of Bombs and Whizz Bangs'. The term 'Whizz Bang' derives from instances where artillery shells are fired from Light or Field Artillery. These shells travel faster than the speed of sound, so soldiers would hear the typical 'whizz' noise of the shell in flight before they heard the 'bang' of the gun being fired. Accordingly 'Whizz Bangs' were much feared because the defending infantry effectively had no warning of incoming high velocity artillery fire compared with that originating from enemy howitzers where the 'bang' was readily heard before the shell arrived. This bombardment resulted in the death of four men and the wounding of a further 10. However, on this occasion, the shelling did not indicate an attack. The Turkish troops remained in ignorance of the evacuation – the fierce defence and counter shelling of the 7th January had apparently convinced them that the Allies were determined to hang on to the beachhead.

Fortunately the Turkish bombardment did not affect the evacuation, which continued as planned, with 'C' Company moving off to Gully Ravine at 11.30, followed an hour later by Battalion HQ. The Grenadiers and Machine Gunners remained to form a covering party while the rest of the battalion set off in small groups during the course of the afternoon. By 17.30 the battalion, less the covering party, proceeded along the seashore to 'W' Beach, where they embarked on the ship SS *Ermine* at 21.15.

The morning of the 9th January saw the battalion's arrival at Mudros, with the Machine Gunners arriving in the afternoon and the Grenadiers on the following day. After a brief period of rest and reinforcement the battalion embarked on the troopship *Simla* on the 19th January, sailing for Alexandria in Egypt. Arriving at Alexandria Harbour on 23rd January, the ship was then diverted to Port Said, which was reached on the 24th, when the battalion disembarked and proceeded to 'Camp A'.

Following the arrival of various reinforcements, the effective strength of the battalion on 8th February was recorded as being 28 Officers, 1 Medical Officer and 729 Other Ranks. From the 9th to the 12th of that month the battalion was engaged in various outpost duties along the Suez Canal before returning to Camp on the 13th February; and it was at this time that Cecil was transferred out.

A diary entry on the 13th February significantly

noted that '13 Other Ranks (Class B) transferred to Details Camp Port Said', and it is highly likely that Cecil was among this particular draft. 'Army Class B' can refer to soldiers who have completed their term of service and are being transferred to the Reserves, but in this particular case it refers to the downgrading of a soldier's fitness level from category 'A' to category 'B'.

The battalion's War Diary covering the period of Cecil's service from September 1915 to January 1916 makes no direct reference at all to any illness or disease afflicting the men. There are a dozen references to various officers either being 'admitted to hospital' or 'sent to the Field Ambulance', but none of these entries make any mention of the officer concerned being wounded in action. Accordingly they must all have been suffering from some disease or another such as dysentery. These scattered references to the circumstances of the battalion's officers give just the merest hint as to what it must have been like for the 'Other Ranks' – the ordinary soldiers such as Cecil.

Dysentery was one of the principal diseases faced by the Army on the Gallipoli Peninsula and was the single largest cause of non-battle casualties, but there were also severe diarrhoea, malaria and enteric fever to contend with. These were all diseases resulting from the insanitary living conditions of the soldiers and were spread by the millions of flies that swarmed everywhere and got into everything. Cecil had also suffered from frostbite in the harsh cold which the troops experienced on the peninsula, although he had fortunately avoided the amputations so often associated with that condition. Health matters for the soldiers were worsened by the monotonous diet of bully beef, hard biscuits, jam and tea, while the limited or largely non-existent facilities for cleaning uniforms meant that their clothing was constantly infested with lice.

Disease was rife throughout the army in Gallipoli, and Cecil's battalion suffered just as much as everyone else. There was also a culture amongst some senior officers who encouraged their men not to report sick but to simply 'soldier on' to offset the acute manpower shortages which the army was experiencing. This approach probably just made things worse. I don't know if Cecil was required to 'soldier on' while afflicted by one of Gallipoli's diseases, but he clearly suffered, and as a result his fitness level was reduced from Class 'A', fit for General Service, to Class 'B', fit for Garrison Service. He was then detailed for return to England.

On the 16th February 1916, after receiving reinforcements and replacements, the battalion embarked on the Troopship *Grampian* and sailed for Kuwait, which it reached on the 28th. Meanwhile Cecil started his journey home on the same day, leaving Alexandria aboard the Hospital Ship *Essequibo* bound for the UK. This ship had previously worked the South America passenger routes, and was named after the Essequibo River in British Guiana (now Guyana). It had been commissioned as a British Hospital Ship in 1915, and was staffed by nurses of the Queen Alexandra's Imperial Military Nursing Service (QAIMNS).

The time taken for ships to sail between the Mediterranean and England varied anywhere between 11 and 22 days, so Cecil probably arrived back in England sometime around the end of February or the early part of March. Landing at Southampton, he was first taken to the nearby Royal Victoria Military Hospital at Netley, where his condition was assessed and any necessary treatment carried out. The hospital was opened in 1863 as Britain's principle military hospital and directly overlooked Southampton Water. A jetty was then added some two years later with the intention of allowing hospital ships to dock and transfer their patients directly into the hospital. Unfortunately this grand idea foundered when it was realised that the water wasn't deep enough, and the ships were in danger of running aground when they tried to reach the jetty. Consequently they were required to dock at Southampton, from where hospital trains then carried their patients on to Netley. The branch line serving the hospital was extended and sidings were added, allowing all the patients to be transferred directly to the wards. The hospital was demolished in 1966 and the grounds were opened in 1980 as the Royal Victoria Country Park. All that remains of the hospital building is the former Chapel, which now serves as a local heritage centre.

Having been discharged from the hospital, Cecil was issued with a travel warrant and allowed to return home on convalescent leave. His journey back to Poole Keynes took him on the Midland & South Western Junction Railway from Southampton to Cirencester's Watermoor Station and would have taken around 2½ hours. After arriving at Cirencester, Cecil then had a walk of six miles or so to his Poole Keynes home.

Cecil's treatment clearly resulted in some improvement to his condition, because his son Dennis Packer, in one of his earliest recollections, used to tell of his Dad's arrival home. Flo was in the cottage preparing a meal of sausage and mash when the children rushed in excitedly to tell her that their Dad was coming down the road. Dashing out of the cottage's front door, Flo screamed in delight as Cecil leapt the garden wall before grabbing her by the waist and spinning her around. She clung to him and they hugged each other before he bent down to gather his sons in his arms in a most happy homecoming.

However her pleasure at seeing Cecil returned after all those months apart must have been tinged with concern at the change in him. The traumas of warfare and his ill health during that wretched autumn and winter on the Gallipoli Peninsula had taken their toll on her husband. He had lost weight and his once tightly-fitting uniform now hung more loosely on him, while his full cheeks were now shrunken. None of this could detract from the sheer joy of his return. Sadly however, this all too brief interlude would prove to be the last occasion on which Cecil was able to spend time with his family.

Leave for soldiers during the war usually lasted for just one week but because Cecil was transferring between units and also required a period of convalescence, his time at home actually lasted for closer to two months. However this may not have all been rest and relaxation, because he was probably attached to the Regiment's Depot and given light duties at the Cirencester recruiting station. Nonetheless he found that the tranquility of Poole Keynes and rural Gloucestershire was a world away from his awful experiences on the Gallipoli Peninsula, and it must have provided a welcome balm to the soul.

However all good things must come to an end and Cecil was soon deemed fit enough to be returned to active duty. Once again he set off in his country's service, but on this occasion to join the 8th (Service) Battalion of the Gloucestershire Regiment in France.

CHAPTER FOUR

THE WESTERN FRONT

Just like Cecil's previous unit in Gallipoli, the 8th was a 'New Army' Battalion created in response to General Kitchener's call for volunteers. It was part of the 19th (Western) Division which had been formed at Bulford, Wiltshire in 1914. Nicknamed 'The Butterfly Division' from the Divisional Sign introduced by its Commanding Officer, General Bridges, early in 1916, the division was undergoing training near Thérouanne in the Pas de Calais area of Northern France. It totaled some 18,000 men divided between three brigades (numbered 56, 57 and 58) with each brigade comprising four infantry battalions. There were also various supporting troops attached both to the brigades and to the division. Cecil's battalion was part of the 57th Brigade alongside the 10th Royal Warwickshire Regiment, the 10th Worcestershire Regiment and the 8th North Staffordshire Regiment.

When Cecil arrived in France he was sent to an Infantry Base Depot located close to Etaples, a small town about 15 miles along the French coast south-west of Boulogne. The depot was one of various holding camps in the area which received men on arrival from England and which were used both for the final training of new recruits and for the retraining (or 'hardening') of veterans such as Cecil before they were posted to an active service unit. Each infantry division had its own Base Depot, so the 19th (Western Division) was supported by No 19 IBD which supplied reinforcements to all the battalions in the division. Each regiment in the division also had its own camp within the Depot.

When he arrived at the camp, Cecil was first sent to the stores to be issued with a rifle and bayonet before being allocated his living quarters which, in common with all the other trainees, consisted of a ten-man tent. He was then required to complete his will, which he dated the 2nd June, thereby indicating the date of his arrival at the Camp, followed by an opportunity to familiarise himself with the camp's layout and facilities before going for his evening meal of bully beef stew. During the evening he was required to attend a lecture regarding the camp's many regulations before being dismissed for the day.

The diary of George Culpitt, serving with the 15th Battalion (London Welsh) Royal Welsh Fusiliers, who was present at the camp shortly before Cecil, records what the training there was like: 'After dinner we fell in and marched to the Ground which was known as the 'Bull Ring'. Passing through the various I.B.D.s and passing the Hospital we got on to the main road to the training area which was some two miles away. On all sides could be seen sand: on the left it stretched away to the sea, while on the right it rose sharply into a large ridge which extended all along the route and was a continuation of the hill on which the Camp stood. Arriving after about 30 minutes marching, hot and perspiring, because it was mid-day and very hot, we turned off the road and... awaited the coming of the sergeant instructors.

'These soon made their appearance, three of them accompanied by an officer, all wearing a wide yellow armband on their sleeves to denote that they were instructors. During the afternoon under the supervision of the sergeants and closely watched by the officer we went through rapid loading, extended order drill, and bayonet fighting and we were much relieved when we finally made our way back to the road, the instructors took their leave and we made tracks for the Depot. The next day found us once again on the Bull Ring but this time in the morning from 8.15am to 12.00 or 1.00pm with a break of half an hour. Bayonet fighting, bombing, and extended order, occupied the morning and we finally arrived back in Camp somewhere about 2.00pm. In this manner the whole of the next ten days with four exceptions were passed. On two days the monotony of training was relieved by a route march.'

The Instructors to whom George refers were known as 'Canaries' on account of their yellow armbands. They later acquired a fearsome reputation, because they were reputed not to have served at the front, and this created a considerable amount of tension between them and veteran soldiers undergoing the sometimes harsh retraining. Conditions at the Depot thus deteriorated in the months after George's description was written and it subsequently became the scene of a serious mutiny in September 1917. The mutiny was prompted by the arrest of a soldier for desertion, although he strenuously denied the charge. News of the event swept through the camp and many of the man's comrades then held a demonstration showing their support for him. This unauthorised act prompted the Military Police to be called and, for some reason, one of them opened fire, killing a soldier and wounding a civilian. This act inflamed the demonstrators, who turned on the MPs and forced them to hurriedly withdraw. At this point the authorities had completely lost control of the situation and for the next three days groups of soldiers roamed the camp searching for the MPs and attacking any hated instructors, while others broke out of the camp and entered the town of Etaples to hold protest meetings.

The demonstrations continued even after the release of the soldier whose arrest had sparked the troubles, but they eventually died down after fresh troops from outside the area, who could be relied upon by the authorities, were brought in to quell the disturbances. Many hundreds of men had been involved in the agitation, but, perhaps in partial recognition of the grievance felt by the troops, and at a time when executions of soldiers were almost commonplace, only one man was actually executed for mutiny. The writer Vera Brittain, who served as a nurse at Etaples during the mutiny, concluded that it 'was due to repressive conditions... and was provoked by the military police'.

Once his training was complete, Cecil was then attached to the 57th Trench Mortar Battery, formed to support the brigade of which his battalion formed part.

The battery had just been established on the 15th June 1916, and was made up of soldiers, like Cecil, who were transferred from the various infantry battalions in the brigade but who continued to retain their parent unit's cap badge. Although I do not know Cecil's reaction to this transfer, I do know that such a move was not always regarded as a welcome posting. The book *Artillery and Trench Mortar Memories* edited by R Whinyates records the diary entry of one soldier sent to a Trench Mortar Battery who wrote: 'We were posted to a unit which we had heard little of at home, and what little we had heard was bad – the Trench Mortars. On hearing our fate our spirits fell considerably as on the way up to the line we had been advised to steer clear of a Trench Mortar Battery. However, we could only make the best of it.'

The Infantry Base Depot has been described as something of a 'melting pot', and it is probable that Cecil was attached to the Trench Mortar Battery direct from the Depot without ever having served with the 8th Battalion as an infantryman. Even if his fitness classification remained at Class B, it is entirely possible that he could have been one of those many men invalided home from the Middle East battle-front whose records were then stamped 'for duty on the Western Front only'. Additionally he had, of course, been employed in the tube cleaning workshop of the GWR, and it is almost certain that the military minds of Cecil's superiors will have linked his work in the GWR with that of operating the tube which formed the primary feature of the trench mortar assembly and concluded that he was thus ideally qualified to work with this new weapon. I think it more than likely therefore that he too felt that he had to 'make the best of it'.

At the start of the war the British Army did not have any trench mortars, although the Germans had three types of Minenwerfer. These weapons soon became a dreadful hazard for those men trying to shelter in the early scratch trenches; the heavy weapon in particular could destroy many yards of trench and cause serious casualties. Accordingly the British authorities decided to design their own mortar, and numerous experiments were undertaken, but many proved to be inaccurate and the bombs mostly exploded prematurely.

The breakthrough came in 1915 with the invention of the 3-inch light mortar designed by Wilfred Stokes, who was the managing director of Ransomes of Ipswich, a company that manufactured cranes. The design was very simple and became the foundation for the 3-inch mortar of the Second World War and the 81mm mortar used by the Army today. The Stokes Mortar had a fixed firing pin, while its bomb was simply a canister of explosive with a percussion fuse. At the base of the bomb was an extension fitted with a blank 12-bore cartridge; this was encircled by horseshoe-shaped secondary charges to give increased range, which was also determined by the angle of the barrel. When the bomb was dropped down the barrel the primer on the cartridge hit the fixed firing pin and ignited, thereby sending the bomb on its way.

According to Mark Adkin, the light mortars were 'easily portable' and could be readily set up and fired from the front-line trenches. As these trenches were seldom more than 800 yards apart, the mortars became 'a deadly and effective addition to trench warfare', hitting enemy positions with shattering effect. Military historian Richard Holmes similarly called them 'cheap, simple and very effective', although they still needed to be operated by skilled crews able to maintain a very high rate of fire, with a number of rounds – perhaps up to nine – in flight at any one time.

By the end of 1915, medium and heavy trench mortars had also been developed. The High Command ordered that these should be manned by the Royal Field Artillery, while the light mortar units would be manned by the infantry. The medium trench mortar batteries formally came under the command of divisional artillery in March 1916, while the light Stokes batteries were removed from infantry battalion control and organised as one trench-mortar company of two four-mortar sections under a Captain in each infantry brigade. At this time the batteries were numbered, and a badge was introduced to identify mortar personnel.

Training in the use of these new weapons was exhaustive, because of the importance attached to them by the military planners seeking ways to break the deadlock on the Western Front. It was hoped that they would be able to play a vital role in achieving ascendancy over the enemy in a variety of situations, both defensive and offensive; from the suppression of an enemy machine-gun, sniper post or other local feature to the coordinated firing of barrages. Accordingly the mortar teams had to be fully trained in these tactics as well as learning how to correctly handle the mortar bombs, which alarmingly retained their tendency to premature explosion.

Serving in a Trench Mortar Battery during the First World War was described to me by Richard Awdry as 'the most dangerous thing you can do', and accidents with these weapons were commonplace. The War Diary for Cecil's battalion towards the end of May recorded that two of the battalion's officers were due to attend a 'demonstration of Stokes Mortars', but the demonstration was cancelled 'owing to an accident'. It was obviously therefore essential for soldiers operating the mortar to work closely together as a team so as to reduce the dangers inherent in the weapon's operation. For example, apart from the risks posed by the basic instability of the mortar bombs, it was found that maintaining the mortar's high rate of fire in the chaos and confusion of a battle could lead to a soldier dropping a fresh bomb into the mortar's barrel before the previous bomb had been fired. Such a mistake could well result in the explosion of both bombs in the barrel, causing the death or serious wounding of the entire mortar crew.

Gordon Corrigan's book *Mud, Blood & Poppycock* also revealed an entirely unforeseen consequence arising from the deployment of some mortar batteries. When being fired from a prepared position, the mortars were sited in a pit, or pits, close to the front line and dug in so that no part of the mortar projected above ground level. These pits however apparently had 'very much the same dimensions as a latrine', and German artillery, firing at targets identified from air photographs which were thought to be mortar positions, often ended up simply shelling the British Army's front line toilets.

Cecil's newly-formed unit also took part in the widespread manoeuvres for companies, brigades and the whole division as the army prepared for the coming offensive. The entire 19th Division moved to a new training area situated east of the Doullens-Amiens Road, which they had reached by the 16th June, with the 57th Brigade and its Trench Mortar Battery being based at Rainneville. Despite this repositioning, the training continued apace in this new location behind the front line which, according to the division's history, resembled 'a vast armed camp'.

An eye witness watching the soldiers moving to take up their positions prior to the offensive wrote to the *Gloucestershire Echo*: 'As we stood, in the shadow of some trees 20 yards from a road which led directly down to the trenches, detachments of our troops could be seen swinging across country in half-companies, companies and battalions. Long before they came close one heard the steady roar of their feet – tramp-tramp, tramp-tramp! And always as they passed they whistled softly in unison. Some whistled 'Tipperary', some whistled 'Come back, my Bonnie, to me', and some, best of all in the place and surroundings, 'La Marseillaise'. As we came back along that road, far behind the front, we saw more companies, more battalions. On the tree-shaded road it was too dark to see them, save only as vague, dark masses against the light background of the highway. One felt their presence... always the steady tramp-tramp, tramp-tramp as they shouldered by, and they were always whistling.' The letter was headlined 'Whistling on the way to death'.

The British Army's campaign on the Somme started on the 1ˢᵗ July 1916, and the day turned out to be a disaster, with an appalling casualty list of nearly 60,000 men, of whom almost 20,000 were killed. The 19th Division's role in the opening battle was to support the assault on the German positions around La Boisselle and to consolidate its capture. La Boisselle was a small village, not unlike Poole Keynes, of 35 houses lying just south of the main Albert-Bapaume Road. It was not an easy place to attack because the German defensive trenches were protected by thick belts of barbed wire and were sited on rising ground which overlooked the British forward positions. This enabled the Germans to clearly see the preparations for any offensive. Having visited those positions myself in 2003, it seemed odd to me that anyone could consider it a good place for an assault. However, and despite the Germans' strength, there was very little choice other than to attack there at that time because of the urgent need to relieve the German pressure on the French, who were suffering grievously in the battles further south around the fortress city of Verdun.

No Man's Land in front of the village was a mass of white chalk craters, piled debris and wire entanglements which formed a death trap for soldiers attempting to cross the dreaded space between the opposing front lines. Even before the massive artillery bombardment which preceded the attack, which had started on the 24th June, the village was little more than a heap of ruins lying amid torn, bare and broken trees blasted almost to stumps. But the walls of the wrecked houses and cottages, although severely damaged, had been formed into machine-gun nests and strong points capable of putting up a formidable resistance.

Viewed with the naked eye from the British lines, La Boisselle seemed to be just a mass of bricks and mortar, strewn here and there with the beams and rafters of tumbled roofs. This led the British commanders to conclude that it was just a rubble heap giving poor protection against an attacking force. But the reality was very different, because the Germans had spent nearly two years turning the village into an immensely strong position, with vast dugouts and shelters, often as much as 30 feet down. These were connected by passages which were proof against the heaviest of British artillery, and where even a small garrison could offer dogged resistance and cause huge casualties amongst the attackers. Mark Adkin quoted a case where a German machine gun post, concealed in a ruined house, was solidly constructed of concrete with 4-inch-thick steel loopholes.

According to 'an onlooker' quoted in Everard Wyrall's

book *The Nineteenth Division 1914-1918*: 'The dawn of the 1ˢᵗ of July seemed calm and sweet. The field on both sides of the line dissembled under a soft mist, above which here and there a high spire or lofty tree just peeped out.' Wyrall then goes on to describe the opening artillery barrage from the British guns, writing that 'at 6.30 there was a sudden roar, an awful rending of the comparative stillness, which left men dazed and with that helpless feeling which comes with an intense thunderclap; the final hour of intense bombardment had begun. All along the line the closely packed trenches showed little movement; all were waiting anxiously for the close of the greatest bombardment of the enemy's defences ever witnessed'.

At 7.30am exactly the artillery suddenly ceased firing and long lines of khaki-clad figures leapt from their trenches and began to move at a steady pace across No Man's Land. Immediately the sharp barking of scores of machine-guns ended the momentary silence and in many places the advancing lines of troops were almost literally swept away. The first waves were followed closely by others, in many places suffering the same terrible fate. The guns dominated No Man's Land and made any attack most difficult. Safe in their deep dugouts, the Germans had waited until the artillery barrage had ceased, then rushed up to the surface, set up their machine-guns and met the first wave of assaulting troops with devastating fire. It didn't matter that the machine-gun emplacements may have been blown away by the artillery barrage; the lip of a shell-hole or crater, or a heap of tumbled bricks was enough shelter to enable them to shoot down the advancing soldiers in their hundreds.

The men attacking La Boisselle succeeded in penetrating part of the enemy's front line but little headway was made elsewhere. By midday progress was limited and no impression at all had been made on the heart of the village. The fighting had been extremely confused and no one could tell how far the troops had got, how much of the enemy's trench system had been captured or where exactly anybody or anything was, though subsequently some of the British dead were later found beyond the village. Yet until La Boisselle was taken further progress was impossible. As the lead divisions had both suffered heavily, the 19th Division was next called upon to join the attack and capture the village. The order was received late in the afternoon of that fateful day, and Cecil's battery was instructed to support an attack on the left side of the village timed to start at 10.30pm.

I cannot imagine what Cecil and his comrades felt at receiving this order. They had spent the day in the reserve trenches and seen the cheerful optimism of the initial attack dissolve into death, destruction and chaos. Although the Trench Mortar Battery was a 'support' unit and wouldn't be in the front line of advancing troops, it nevertheless had to follow them closely to provide local artillery support with their mortars to help overcome the enemy strong points and machine-gun nests. Cecil and the others could therefore be forgiven for fearing that they were about to share the same frightful fate as those earlier attackers.

However, as they attempted to move forward, they found that the trench systems in front of them were blocked by groups of stretcher-bearers, wounded men and miscellaneous crowds of troops resulting from the day's confused fighting. Parties of men were going up to the front line, others were coming back, and it proved to be utterly impossible for the men of the 57th Brigade and their supporting units to get into their attack positions. Their plan of attack was therefore abandoned and the men had to remain where they were, to spend an awful night wondering what was in store for them the next day.

By dawn on the 2nd July, under a clear blue sky, the 57th Brigade found itself occupying front line trenches opposite La Boisselle but with no orders to advance. As the temperature rose to 75deg F the brigade remained where they were while attacks were carried out at other points along the line. Indeed, it wasn't until the early hours of the morning, 3.15 am on the 3rd July, that the brigade was eventually ordered into action. Advancing over ground still littered with the dead and dying of the previous attacks, the infantry fought their way into the village. They were supported in this by the mortar battery crews, who were manoeuvring their heavy equipment around the battlefield and aiding the suppression of enemy defensive fortifications while managing, at the same time, to maintain the supply of ammunition which the mortars quickly consumed. In a report after the battle it was noted that the mortars' 'mobility allowed of their being carried forward in spite of the difficulties of the ground', while the report's author (Major General John Headlam) further wrote, 'I myself saw two batteries that they had been so brought forward and ascertained that they had been able to get up several hundred rounds'.

The Germans were still resisting strongly, but their defences had been weakened by the earlier attacks, and by the time the outskirts of the village were secured, about 100 or so Germans had surrendered. Finally, at 8.10am, Divisional HQ was informed that the village had been captured apart from some snipers lurking in the dugouts and ruins. However, about twenty minutes later, a fierce German counter-attack was launched leading to what was described as 'probably the most intense fighting the division had up to that period experienced'. The ferocity of this attack forced the British back, and the position by about 12.30pm had become desperate, particularly for the men of the 57th Brigade who held a hedge line where very hard fighting took place. The value of the close support provided by the likes of Cecil's Trench Mortar Battery certainly proved its worth at this time because, had the line been overrun, the enemy could well have recaptured the whole village. Most of the battalion commanders were either killed or wounded during this ferocious battle but, under the unified command of Lt Col Adrian Carton de Wiart of the 8th Gloucesters, they held on and repulsed the counter-attack.

Lt Colonel (later Lt General) Carton de Wiart, who had lost his left eye fighting with the Camel Corps in Somaliland in 1914, and had his left hand amputated while serving with the 4th Dragoon Guards at Ypres in 1915, was awarded the VC for his bravery and leadership during the battle at La Boisselle. Described as 'truly exceptional and courageous', de Wiart was an accomplished leader of men. Dr Anthony Clayton, a former senior lecturer at Sandhurst, said that de Wiart 'commanded a personal respect among the men he led in battle. Soldiers could see that he was a man who had been where he was asking them to go.' Carton de Wiart served his country again in the Second World War, and lived to the ripe old age of 83 before passing away in June 1963.

Although the 57th Brigade still occupied their positions, they were unable to advance against the enemy gathered in front of them. The divisional history later recorded that 'By the evening of 3rd July the whole of La Boisselle was not yet in our hands. In the eastern end several pockets of Germans still held out, offering the stoutest resistance, while sporadic bombing continued throughout the night of the 3rd/4th July.'

At 8.30am on the 4th July, under an overcast sky, the final attack was launched against the German positions. Once again there was fearsome fighting against determined German resistance, particularly around a group of four houses and adjacent shell-holes manned by machine-gunners. These were eventually cleared under mortar fire from Cecil's battery and at the point of the bayonet, and by 3pm, the whole of La Boisselle had been captured, although sporadic shell-fire and sniping continued afterwards. Following its capture the village was said to be 'unrecognisable as ever having been the habitation of human beings.' The 19th Division's Memorial now stands in the middle of the village, which, along with the nearby hamlet of Ovillers, was 'adopted' by the city of Gloucester during the 1920s. This act symbolised the strong link between that sector of the Somme battlefield and the number of men from the Glosters who fell there in its liberation and subsequent defence.

At 9pm on the 5th July the brigade began to pull back to Albert, being relieved by fresh troops. This move was completed by 12.30am, although Cecil's Trench Mortar Battery and the Machine Gun Company were required to remain in the village providing fire cover for the incoming troops. Later that morning, after being subsequently withdrawn, they reached Albert, where the 57th Brigade was held in reserve while other units were in action. The division's history later recorded that the capture of La Boisselle owed much to inter-unit co-operation (including that between infantry and trench mortar crews) which it stated was 'as near perfect as human nature could make it.' Then, on the 10th July, the whole of the division marched three miles back down the road to Millencourt, where the men could rest, relax, refresh and undergo retraining for the next stage in the campaign.

I do hope that this retraining which Cecil and the other soldiers of the brigade had to undertake was of more use than that described by Frederic Manning in his book *The Middle Parts of Fortune*. Although the book is a work of fiction, originally published in 1929, Manning did serve during the campaigns in this part of France at the same time as Cecil, and many of the incidents in the book are based on actual events. In it he describes an attack training exercise where the brigade was formed up in open countryside with, to their front, a mass of tapes showing the layout of the trenches to be attacked. Manning writes: 'The files of men moved forward slowly, and when they reached the tapes, followed the paths assigned to them with an admirable precision. Their formations were not broken up or depleted by any hostile barrage, the ground was not pitted by craters, their advance was not impeded by any uncut wire. Everything went according to plan. It was a triumph of staff work'. But of course, it bore no relation whatsoever to the fury, chaos and horror that the men would face in a real attack.

When their rest and retraining period ended on the 19th July, the 57th Brigade marched seven miles from Millencourt to a bivouac area at Fricourt, where they spent the night before continuing for a further four miles to take up front-line positions in the vicinity of the village of Bazentin le Petit. However the 'front line' there had only recently been captured and the original trenches were largely destroyed by artillery fire, so a clear trench line did not exist. The 'line' was held by a combination of short lengths of trench, and holes wherever soldiers could dig themselves in. The ground in the locality was described as being 'smashed beyond recognition.' The divisional history also noted that close to the nearby High Wood 'lay a number of dead horses which stank so much that passing them was almost more unpleasant than passing over heavily-shelled ground.'

Having occupied these somewhat precarious positions, Cecil and every other man in the brigade were then immediately employed working hard to improve the defences and create fresh trench systems. German shell-fire during this time was heavy, and snipers were everywhere; the continual crash of explosions and crack of rifle fire regularly causing Cecil and the others to stop their work as they dived for cover. This incessant enemy fire made movement by day very difficult and dangerous, and is recorded as having 'tried the endurance of the troops to the utmost' – a description which seems to me to be yet another case of classic British understatement.

The 19th Division moved forward to attack the German trenches at 12.30am on the 23rd July. The infantry of 57 Brigade, supported by its Trench Mortar Battery, advanced along their frontage to within 75 yards of the German trenches but were halted by heavy machine-gun fire. Unable to press home their advance, they gradually pulled back to their start-line by 6.55am. Although this retirement signalled the end of the day's attack, it didn't provide a break for the men because they were immediately put to work on further strengthening their defences and preparing for their next attack. This eventually took place on the 30th July, when a section of the German trench was captured and occupied while repeated counter-attacks by the Germans were successfully resisted and the position was consolidated. The brigade was eventually relieved on the 31st July by other units and was then able to pull back to its reserve positions.

The beginning of August saw the 19th Division withdrawn from the Somme sector entirely and sent to occupy trenches to the south-east of Ypres. This was considered by the Army's senior officers to be a comparatively quiet part of the line where Cecil and his comrades would have some small opportunity to recover from the strenuous and fearsome days of July. Travelling by train, the troops arrived at Bailleul and occupied the front-line trenches there during the night of 7th/8th August. Coincidentally, Cecil's new station was only just over eight miles from where his brother-in-law, John Davis, had been killed the previous year.

This new location may well have been regarded by those anonymous officers as being quieter than the Somme, but it certainly wasn't a rest area, and it was still very dangerous – men were routinely being killed and wounded by German machine-gun fire, sniping and shelling. The soldiers were also constantly engaged in maintaining and repairing the trenches, while regular patrols were sent out to examine the enemy's wire and trench positions. Cecil's battery was also continually in action mortaring the German lines. For example the War Diary of the 8th Glosters on the 11th August recorded: 'Very quiet except from 4.30 to 5.30pm when the enemy was active with bombs and rifle grenades on our front line and Minenwerfer bombs and trench mortars on our supports. Our Stokes mortars and 18pdrs replied.' Again, on the 21st, the diary noted: 'Our artillery and Trench Mortars heavily bombarded enemy reserve and support trenches'.

On the 6th September the entire division was moved to occupy fresh positions between the Lys and Douvre Rivers. Raids and fights in No Man's Land were a particular feature of this sector of the front and Cecil's battery was often used to provide supporting mortar fire to cover the raiding soldiers. Notwithstanding all of this activity, the divisional history somewhat laconically commented that 'During the period – roughly two months – spent away from the Somme, there is little of outstanding importance to record.'

When not in action operating the mortar or called upon to do other work, Cecil was able to take shelter in a dugout which will also have often provided the setting for his meals and sleeping accommodation. Dugouts had begun to appear along the front during the course of 1915 and were established to protect soldiers from the effects of shelling. They were used to house all types of front-line headquarters as well as providing shelter for troops such as mortar crews who were not permanently required on the firing line. A typical dugout was formed by digging a large deep pit with sloping access which could later be formed into stairs; it was then roofed over with timber, or perhaps concrete, and thickly covered in earth. Despite the dangers of flooding or collapse, these often rudimentary shelters could then be developed over time to provide extensive and, in many cases, reasonably secure accommodation.

The large dugouts almost always led off from the support or reserve trenches, and a Company Sergeant Major on the Somme in 1916 described his dugout as being 'the best I have ever been in.' He continued by saying that 'the dugout is parted in three – one part is for the telephone and operators, officers' servants and trench mortar batteries attached. The centre part is for the Officers and the third part is for the stretcher-bearers, company and platoon orderlies, sanitary men and myself.'

It may seem strange, even in those times, that officers should have 'servants' in the middle of a war zone, but the servant was more commonly known as an officer's 'batman'. He was usually a volunteer on extra duty paid for by the officer, and was responsible for the officer's clothing and kit, and also for preparing and serving meals. He acted as a bodyguard when in the trenches and carried his officers' personal weapon when the officer undertook his various duties as platoon, company or battalion commander.

Starting on the night of 4th/5th October the division began its return to the Somme, and by the 22nd of the month Cecil and his comrades in the brigade's Trench Mortar Battery were occupying positions south of the River Ancre, in front of which was the village of Grandcourt. Behind them and standing high on a ridge were the shattered ruins of Thiepval village, which is now the site of the massive Thiepval Memorial designed by Sir Edwin Lutyens and unveiled in 1932. It contains the names of 72,195 soldiers killed in the battles of the Somme between 1915 and 1918 who have no known grave.

On the 23rd October the 19th Division received its first order to attack northwards towards Grandcourt and the line of the River Ancre, but shortly afterwards the attack was postponed due to bad weather – an altogether too familiar situation throughout this part of the campaign, and one that would constantly bedevil even the best-laid battle plans. This situation is probably best illustrated by the divisional history, which at the time reported: 'Winter had set in on the Somme, and the low-lying country in the Ancre valley had begun to fill with water, the heavy rains turning trenches into waterways and the ground round about into spongy morasses. As the days grew shorter and greyer the desolation became more pronounced. The roads were thick with mud, the tracks across country mere mud walks and the pock-marked ground, churned up by shells of all calibre, exuded water which filled the shell-holes and polluted the air with nauseating smells'.

This dramatic change in conditions has also made it rather more difficult to follow Cecil's role in the battle of the Ancre, because his unit's tactics would almost certainly have changed from those employed during the summer battles. During that time the firm ground will have allowed the men of the mortar battery to move their equipment around the battlefield with comparative ease and as required in support of the infantry, so the infantry's story is also essentially the story of the mortar crews. But the increasingly muddy conditions on the Ancre will have made any movement with bulky equipment extremely difficult, if not virtually impossible. I therefore think it almost certain that Cecil's Trench Mortar Battery will have played a much more static role than had been the case previously.

Following a small improvement in the weather conditions, fresh preparations were made for a renewed offensive which involved a certain shuffling and moving around of units along the front line. The opening gambit of this attack took place on the 13th November but didn't involve Cecil's battery or any of the units of 57 Brigade. The attack was successful and the targeted enemy positions were captured. The 57th Brigade remained a bystander until they were brought into action for the main offensive on the 18th November. However the weather drastically worsened late on the night of the 17th and seriously affected their attack. This was launched at 6.10am across the entire divisional front and involved every unit including the Trench Mortar Batteries, but it followed an overnight snowfall and the attack began in whirling sleet which later changed to rain. Visibility at the start was severely limited by the sleet, and features on the ground were indistinguishable from each other because they were all covered in snow.

Some units suffered heavy casualties when they were raked by machine-gun fire as they were stopped by uncut barbed wire, although the 8th Glosters did succeed in entering the south-western end of Grandcourt. However the attack's almost universal lack of success, in appalling conditions, and with one battalion being almost entirely lost, led to the abandonment of offensive operations for the winter. The remnants of the 8th Gloucesters were therefore withdrawn from the positions they had captured and a line about 1,000 yds further back was consolidated. This enabled a ferocious German counter-attack in chilling rain to be beaten off during the course of following morning.

The 19th Division was then relieved by another division during the period of the 20th to 23rd November. This allowed the 57th Brigade to move into quarters some 26 miles away at Gezaincourt near Doullens, where the men could at last have a decent hot meal and a good wash and clean themselves of the glutinous mud. The appalling conditions which Cecil and the other soldiers endured during this part of the campaign are perhaps best described in the divisional history:

'The story of the Battle of the Ancre, 1916, makes dismal reading: it could not be otherwise seeing the terrible conditions under which the attack took place. No troops in the world could have advanced more gallantly to the attack, but no troops in the world could have kept direction in the midst of a snow storm, intense darkness, and over ground that was thick in mud, pock-marked with shell-holes and with little or nothing to guide them to their objectives. Not since the 19th Division had arrived in France had such appalling conditions been experienced. The grimness of the Ancre battlefield became graven on the mind – the cold, the rain and snow, the ghastly gloomy country, the ceaseless shell-fire, the clinging mud into which men and horses sank sometimes with fatal results. All units suffered alike. Every round of artillery fired had to be carried up by pack transport, and the poor animals often collapsed and sank dead into the all-enveloping mud. The Royal Army Medical Corps, in bringing back wounded men, had a terrible time; the Sappers, the Pioneers, all seemed to wallow in mud.'

On the 4th December Cecil's battery received orders to move a further two miles or so to Beauval, where a Mortar Training School had been established, although the specific tasks of the soldiers in the battery are not recorded. The War Diary for the 57th Infantry Brigade HQ for the early part of December simply records that members of the brigade were engaged in 'training', while the War Diary for the 8th Glosters notes that the training included such matters as 'arms drill', 'bayonet fighting' and 'musketry'. There must also have been training carried out in the tactics and use of trench mortars, although these activities are not mentioned in the diaries. Sporting pursuits had their part to play in the training programme as well, and on the 10th December a football match was held between the Glosters and the 10th Battalion Worcestershire Regiment which the Glosters lost by three goals to one.

Unfortunately however, the trench mortar rounds, even when just being used for training, remained dangerously temperamental. On the 13th December 1916, Cecil was handling a mortar round when it exploded, and he was killed.

Cecil's death was reported back home in Cirencester's local newspaper, the *Wilts and Gloucestershire Standard*, on the 20th January 1917, and the report merits repeating:

'News has been received of the death in France of Private C T Packer, the Gloucestershire Regiment, attached to the Trench Mortar Battalion, third son of Mr T Packer, labourer of Poole Keynes, now of Oaksey, and son-in-law of Mr F Davis of Poole Keynes. The deceased, who leaves a widow and five children, served in the Gallipoli Peninsula, and afterwards in France, taking part in the recent heavy fighting in connection with the offensive on the Western Front, being afterwards accidentally killed at one of the trench mortar schools. The Captain commanding his battery, writing to Mrs Packer to express his deep sympathy, and stating where the deceased is buried, says: "He was liked by all the men of the battery, and I personally can say I have never met a finer man." One of his comrades, Private F Pottinger, wrote to Mrs Packer saying that her husband was killed on December 13, adding: "He was liked by everyone in the battery and the Captain thought such a lot of him... I have lost my best mate. I feel sorry for you and his children, as he was always on about his children... I am sending a post card that came with a parcel for your husband. It had been broken open and repacked when I received it. There were socks, gloves and a scarf in it when I received it." Lance-Corporal Toft writes: "I was at the school when the accident happened. I can tell you he did not suffer at all... He was a good man and a brave man, and I feel sorry to my heart. I often think of him and pray for him."

Cecil's War service entitled him to three medals – the 1914-15 Star, the British War Medal and the Victory Medal. His death in the war also entitled his family to be presented with the Memorial Medallion. Sadly all of these items seem to have since been lost.

The **1914 – 1915 Star** was awarded to those who saw

service in any theatre of war between 5ᵗʰ August 1914 and 31ˢᵗ December 1915. The medal is bronze with the recipient's number, rank and unit carved on the reverse. Its award automatically entitled the recipient to the British War Medal and the Victory Medal.

The **British War Medal** was the standard silver war medal for the First World War. The ribbon colours are not supposed to have any significance. The medal shows the head of King George V on the obverse, while the reverse depicts a naked warrior on horseback trampling the Arms of the Central Powers and the emblems of death.

The **Victory Medal** is a bronze gilt-washed medal showing a winged Victory on the obverse, with the slogan 'The Great War For Civilisation 1914-1919' on the reverse. The rainbow colours on the ribbon applied to all Allied medals, and it is sometimes known as 'the Allied War Medal'. The Victory Medal is never worn by itself, but always in conjunction with at least the British War Medal or other 1914-1918 Awards.

Collectively the three medals were commonly called 'Pip, Squeak and Wilfred' after popular cartoon characters of the time.

The **Memorial Medallion** was issued after the war to the next-of-kin of all British and Empire service personnel who were killed as a result of the war. The medallion was made of bronze and popularly known as the 'Death Penny' or the 'Dead Man's Penny' because of its similarity to the somewhat smaller one-penny coin then in circulation. The Medallion showed an image of Britannia holding a trident and standing with a lion, while her outstretched left hand holds an oak wreath above a rectangular tablet bearing the deceased's name in raised letters. The rank of the deceased is not shown, to avoid any distinction being made regarding an individual's sacrifice. Two dolphins swim around Britannia, symbolising Britain's sea power, and at the bottom a second lion is shown tearing apart the German eagle. Circling this picture are the words (in capital letters): 'HE DIED FOR FREEDOM AND HONOUR'. The reverse of the medallion was blank.

POSTSCRIPT

It seems that around the time that Cecil was sent to France, or shortly thereafter, Flo was required to move out of her rented home at 105 Poole Keynes. Cecil had completed his Army Will on the 2nd July 1916, making Flo his beneficiary and describing her address by then as being no. 108 Poole Keynes. This was one of a pair of cottages situated on the opposite side of the road to the Poole Keynes school building, which have since been merged. It was then also larger than no. 105, being shown on the 1911 census as having four rooms. At that time it was occupied by Farm Carter William Willavoys and his family of three adults and three children.

This change of home was likely to have been brought about by the need to fill Cecil's role of shepherd at Glebe Farm and to provide accommodation for his replacement, and no. 105 was probably required for this purpose. However people in the village would not have wished to see Flo and her children made homeless, so the Reverend Wells doubtless arranged for her to move into no. 108, which had recently become vacant.

The duration of Flo's stay at 108 is not known, but, probably around the time she was found to be expecting another child, or perhaps a little later, she moved to live with her parents at their Oakwell Cottage, no. 117 Poole Keynes. The precise date of Flo's arrival is not recorded, but I think some of the individuals listed as being there at the time of the 1911 census must surely have moved on by then. It was an invariable practice of the period for some children in large families to be boarded out with relatives who had fewer children, or to leave home early to serve as apprentices or domestic servants, and without those departures I don't think the cottage could have coped with all of them as well as the arrival of a pregnant Flo and her family.

Life was clearly not easy for Flo with Cecil away serving at the front while she had four children to look after as well as having to cope with the changes of home. However she did have a very supportive family in addition to many friends in the village, and I think she was also blessed with considerable strength of character. She was also considered to be something of a psychic, having a talent for clairvoyance and an ability to 'read' tea leaves. Indeed this seems to have been something of a family trait, because her younger brother Charles later became a medium/faith healer.

This family aptitude may well have had something to do with a strange occurrence when Flo received the news of Cecil's death. Family legend clearly records that at the exact time that she cried out in shock while reading the telegram bringing the awful news, the tall grandfather clock in the cottage's living room stopped – just like the grandfather clock in the 19th Century song. Although unlike that particular clock, this one is said to have later mysteriously restarted of its own accord.

The cruel blow of Cecil's death must have hit Flo particularly hard, coming as it did barely 24 months after the death of her younger brother. Her pregnancy was well advanced when she received the sad news, and the terrible shock of losing her beloved husband caused her go into early labour. Flo's fifth son, named Cecil in honour and memory of his father, was then born on the 4th January 1917, and his premature birth ironically resulted in him sharing the same birthday as his older brother Leslie.

On the morning of the 7th January, a mere three days after Cecil was born, Flo made her way to the Cirencester Registry Office to register his birth. Once there she recorded his full name as 'Cecil Charles Packer', while sadly noting at the same time that her husband Cecil Thomas Packer, the father of the child, was now 'deceased'.

Flo's next address after moving on from her parents' cottage was shown on Cecil's Army pension records for July 1917 as being no. 112 Poole Keynes. This was one of a pair of cottages opposite West End Farm and a short distance from Oakwell on the road to the village; it was described on the 1911 census as a three-room property, being then occupied by the family of C.J. Hicks, a farm labourer. However, by the time of the war's end, around 1918/1919, Flo had finally returned to live in her original village home at no. 105.

During the course of the inevitable upheavals resulting from these various changes of home, Flo's eldest son Frank, who was aged nine by June 1917, had been sent to stay with his grandparents, Thomas and Ellen Packer, who were by that time living in Oaksey. Dennis's daughter, Maureen Rose, remembered her uncle Frank telling her of the time that he spent in Oaksey with his grandparents, whom he described as being 'very strict'. He was required to read the Bible on

Sundays in addition to attending the local church on a day that was wonderfully described by Maureen as being 'very much a day of Sunday attire and religion'. She went on to say that Frank had found life there to be 'quite hard but he loved to visit his mother'.

Thomas and Ellen had probably moved to Oaksey at some point during 1916, perhaps when Thomas was no longer able to continue working at Lower Farm and had to leave his tied cottage. They are both described as being 'of Oaksey' in the January 1917 newspaper report of Cecil's death, while the Oaksey Electoral Registers for 1918 and the autumn of 1919 both record them as residing in the village at a property described as being 'by Brook Cottage'. They remained at that address until late 1919 or early 1920 when the Crudwell Electoral Register shows them to be finally living at Eastcourt, a small settlement between Oaksey and Crudwell.

It was at Eastcourt, on the 8th September 1924, that Ellen died and was buried three days later in Crudwell churchyard. Thomas survived her by a little over five months before dying at the home of his daughter Sarah and son-in-law Ernest Musty in Little Faringdon, Berkshire, on the 25th February 1925, being buried in Crudwell on the 5th March. I have attempted to locate their graves, but without success. The very helpful Crudwell Churchwarden, Cathy Butcher, told me that, sadly, the church does not have any records relating to the location of unmarked graves such as those for Thomas and Ellen. Nonetheless I do hope they were buried close to each other.

There was no provision for the payment of a widow's pension from Cecil's work with the GWR or, indeed, from his work on the farm, but Flo did of course receive a widow's pension from the Army. This was paid at a weekly rate of 13/9d starting in July 1917 with additional, graduated, payments for each of her dependants: she received 5/- for the first son (Frank), 4/2d for the second son (Cecil John), 3/4d for the third son (Dennis), and 2/6d each for the fourth and fifth sons (Leslie & Cecil Charles). The pension payments for the boys stopped when they reached 16 years of age, and Flo was warned that payment of her widow's pension would also stop if and when she remarried.

These various payments gave Flo a total pension income of 31/3d per week, which may seem generous in comparison with Cecil's pre-war wages. However any direct comparison is difficult because of the severe inflation experienced during the war, which averaged 17.2% between 1915 and 1920. Accordingly Flo took on a variety of jobs in order to supplement her pension and to help provide for her family. Maureen told me that her Granny 'could do anything. She took in washing or walked miles to do sewing for people; the boys were devoted to her'. Maureen said that Flo also suffered from diabetes mellitus and was quite often very ill, although she further described her as 'a poet, happy and gregarious.' Many years later Dennis's son Edward did some work for a local lady called Mrs Selwyn, who described Flo as 'the best woman I've ever met'.

In February 1920 the *Wilts & Glos Standard* reported that the Reverend Wells of Poole Keynes had received permission to 'to erect in the Parish Church on the north wall of the nave a brass tablet to commemorate the names of the fallen soldiers in the Great War'. The memorial contains seven names, including that of 31-year-old Cecil T Packer and his 22-year-old brother-in-law Francis J Davis, and it is a list that has been correctly described as being 'a heavy toll for a village of 140 inhabitants.' The memorial tablet was designed and manufactured by a company founded by William Morris (1834-1896), and the newspaper report went on to note that its cost 'will be defrayed by the Parishioners.' William Morris was famous for his 'Arts and Crafts' fabric and wallpaper designs between 1880 and 1910, and the leaves decorating each corner of the memorial are typical of that style.

The unveiling of the memorial took place on Wednesday the 28th April 1920 during a service in the church which was described in the *Wilts and Gloucestershire Standard* as 'an auspicious event in the history of the tiny and remote parish of Poole Keynes'. The Rector noted that the church was 'full of people', while the seating close to the memorial was reserved for the servicemen's relatives, who, in the words of the newspaper reporter, 'sorrowed the loss of their loved ones.' Flo sat there with her family mourning the loss of both her husband and brother, and she must have experienced a poignant moment indeed as the memorial was unveiled. This was done by the Hon Mrs John Biddulph of Kemble House, who was reportedly 'filled with deepest sympathy' for those who were bereaved. The unveiling was followed by the dedication of the memorial in a service conducted by the Reverend Wells which was described by the newspaper as being 'simple yet beautiful.'

Some 18 months later, in October 1921, Flo's mother Sarah died at Oakwell and was buried in Oaksey. Flo's father, widower Frank Davis, then remarried in Stroud on the 3rd May 1922. His address on the Marriage Certificate is simply shown as 'Poole Keynes', indicating that he was still living at no. 117. His new wife was a widow, Elizabeth Bishop of Brimscombe, near Stroud, who was more popularly known as 'Ginny' and was some 20 years younger than him.

It was around this time that Flo left Poole Keynes and moved to a council house in Kemble. The Electoral Register shows Florence Annie Packer living at 105 Poole Keynes in the 1921 autumn edition, but by the spring of 1922 the Register shows her to be living at the 'RD Council Cottage' in Kemble. The house was later known as no. 5 Council Houses, and is located in Windmill Road. It was while she was living there that her second-born son, 17-year-old Cecil John (Jack), who was a 'motor engineer', died in Cirencester's Memorial Hospital on the 5th March 1927. His brothers, Frank and Dennis, had walked the five miles from Kemble to the hospital to visit him, but he passed away just before they arrived. This left them with the heartbreaking task of walking all the way back to Kemble to break the sad news to their mother. Five days later Jack was buried in Poole Keynes churchyard, but Flo could not afford a stone, so the grave is unmarked.

Shortly thereafter, Flo's father Frank and stepmother Ginny moved in to live with her, being shown as living at the council house on the 1928 and subsequent editions of the Electoral Register. Frank then died on the 21st November 1931, and his widow subsequently remarried in late 1947, moving away to live in Edmonton, north London.

Flo then married widower William John Strange at

Kemble on the 30th July 1932. William was described on the Marriage Certificate as an 'Engine Man GWR,' and he lived at no. 4 Railway Cottages, close to Kemble Station. These stone-built cottages, overlooking the branch line to Cirencester, had been constructed by the GWR in the late 19th Century to provide accommodation for their many employees, and families, based in the village. Maureen said 'Granny married when the boys were grown up' and described William as 'strict but good to Granny. They lived at the council house in Kemble'.

Flo's remarriage was later followed by the marriages of her and Cecil's surviving sons. Frank was the first, when he married Elizabeth Wood in 1935, then Dennis married Helen Harris in 1936, Cecil Charles married Monica Ravenhill in 1940, and finally Leslie married Margaret Reckherling in 1947.

After their wedding Flo and William Strange lived for a while in Watermoor Road, Cirencester, where the 1939 Register shows them in September of that year to be living at no. 149. William is described as a 'Retired Boilerman', while Flo is said to be engaged in 'Unpaid Domestic Duties'. Following the marriage of Cecil Charles to Monica at the beginning of 1940, Flo and William moved to live with them in Thornbury, a market town to the north of Bristol. They lived there in Silver Street until William's death from pneumonia in the early part of 1947. Flo then moved back to Wiltshire, probably in about 1949, because the Electoral Register shows her that year living at Ivy Cottage, Eastcourt. Maureen said that Flo became 'a companion/carer to Miss Sutton in Eastcourt who was disabled and unable to walk'. Flo also 'cleaned and helped the two Cook boys' – Fred and Bill – who worked on Oatridge Farm and lived nearby in a cottage at Flintham Hill, which is on the road from Eastcourt to Oaksey. By 1951 Flo was also living at Flintham Hill as a live-in housekeeper to the Cook brothers, and she then married Fred Cook on the 27th September 1952. Fred was 15 years younger than Flo, but Maureen described him as 'a kind gentleman.'

Flo, Fred and Bill Cook continued to share the Flintham Hill cottage until the brothers retired from their work on the farm, following which all three moved to live in a council house just a couple of miles away at 28 Tuners Lane in Crudwell. This house was comparatively new, having been built in 1950, and it was large enough to allow Flo's stepmother Ginny to come and live there when she moved back to Wiltshire following the death of her third husband in late 1960. Maureen said 'I remember her well. She was softly spoken and very pleasant. She and Granny were much the same age and got on well. They were great friends'. The four of them lived in Tuners Lane until Flo died in

Watermoor Hospital, Cirencester on the 9th March 1966, followed two months later by Fred, who died in Bristol Royal Infirmary. Flo and Fred were both buried in Crudwell churchyard, although, as with others before them, their graves sadly have no stone.

CONCLUSION

I didn't really know what I would find when I started the detailed research of Cecil's life, but in putting his story into words I have discovered a quite extraordinary man whose comparatively short life encompassed a range of hugely different undertakings. He was a farm labourer, a factory labourer, a shepherd and a soldier, and as such, he exhibited those characteristics of men from the villages which were held in such high esteem by Alfred Williams. He had surely proven himself to be, in Williams' words, 'fresh and tractable, open to receive new ideas and impressions of things'.

However, and above all, I also discovered a family

man who still had the courage to answer his country's call in time of war and to leave behind all those that he held dear. Richard Awdry sadly passed away while I was conducting my research, but his widow, Gill, very kindly allowed me access to Richard's notes on the names of the men listed on the Poole Keynes War Memorial. Writing of Cecil's time in what he described as 'some of the most appalling battlefields of the Great War, at Gallipoli and on the Somme', Richard rightly concluded that Cecil was indeed 'a brave and gallant man'.

Having expressed the hope in the Introduction that I thought Cecil's story needed to be known by a much wider audience, I think this work has now helped to achieve that aim. However the writing of Cecil's story has additionally revealed another extraordinary individual – his wife Flo, who was so unhappily widowed and left with five boys under the age of nine to care for. Nonetheless, Poole Keynes was then, indeed I think it still is, a closely-knit community, and it was this closeness that must surely have helped her to keep the family together in those dark and difficult years after Cecil was killed.

Gordon Corrigan concluded his book on the First World War with the statement: 'In what those men did, and in how they did it, we should feel pride today'. He could well have been writing about the pride we should all feel for the sacrifice of Cecil Thomas Packer, to which I add the pride that we should also feel for the fortitude and forbearance of his wife and widow, Florence Annie Packer.

BIBLIOGRAPHY
& SOURCES

- Adkin, Mark. 'The Western Front Companion'. Aurum Press 2013

- Baily & Woods Cirencester Directory 1908-1911.

- Bartlett, Keith. 'Battlefront: Somme. Facsimile Documents Series.' Public Record Office. 2002.

- Beckett Ian F W. 'Discovering English County Regiments'. Shire Publications 2003.

- Brann, Christian (Ed). 'Kemble Ewen and Poole Keynes'. Collectors Books Ltd 1992.

- Bray, Nigel. 'The Cirencester Branch.' The Oakwood Press 1998.

- Brill, Edith. 'Life and Tradition on the Cotswolds'. J M Dent & Sons Ltd 1973.

- Brown, Jonathan. 'Shepherds and Shepherding'. Shire Publications 2013.

- Bryan, Tim. 'The Golden Age of the Great Western Railway.' Patrick Stephens Ltd 1992.

- Burderop Park Training College. 'Work Wages and Pastimes. Swindon 1800 – 1950'. Undated.

- Clark, Christopher. 'The Sleepwalkers. How Europe Went to War in 1914'. Penguin Books 2013.

- Corrigan, Gordon. 'Mud, Blood and Poppycock. Britain and the First World War.' Cassell 2003

- Cuss HW John. 'The Valley of the Upper Thames'. Robert Hale 1998.

- Glidden, Gerald. 'The Battle of the Somme - A topographical History.' Sutton Publishing 1987.

- Gloucestershire Archives: File Refs: G/CI/159/17 (Rate book for Poole Keynes 1918 & 1920-1925); GDR/F1/1/1920/19 (Brass Tablet as War Memorial); P251 CW 2/1 & 2/2 (Churchwarden's and Charity Accounts); P251 IN 1/6 (Transcript of the Poole Keynes Parish Registers); P251 IN 1/7 (Register of Services for Poole Keynes); P251 OV 8/6 (Poole Keynes Rate Book 1889/90); P251 VE 2/1 (Poole Keynes Parish & Charity Records 1892-1915); Q/RER/1918 – 1935 (Various Electoral Registers for the Parishes of Poole Keynes & Kemble).

- Great Western Railway 'Timetables 1902 & 1932'. GWR.

- Hart, George. 'Edgar Corble – Primus In Urbe.' Old Masonians Gazette 2015.

- Haythornthwaite, Philip. 'The World War 1 Source Book'. Cassell 1992.

- Hey, David (Ed). 'The Oxford Companion to Local and Family History'. OUP 1995.

- Holmes, Richard. 'Tommy'. Harper Collins 2004.

- Huxley, Elspeth. 'Gallipot Eyes - A Wiltshire Diary'. Weidenfeld & Nicholson 1976.

- James, Brig E A. OBE TD 'British Regiments 1914 - 1918'. Naval & Military Press 1978.

- Kelly's 'Gloucestershire Directory' 1906.

- Mallinson, Allan. '1914 Fight the Good Fight.' Bantam Press 2014.

- Matheson, Rosa. 'Railway Voices 'Inside' Swindon Works'. The History Press 2008

- McCarthy, Chris. 'The Somme - The Day-by-day Account'. Brockhampton Press 1998.

- Middlebrook, Martin. 'Your Country Needs You'. Pen & Sword Books Ltd 2000.

- Moorehead, Alan, 'Gallipoli'. Illustrated Edition. Macmillan 1975.

- National Archives: File Refs: WO 25/3536 (Embarkation Returns Home for Abroad July – Sept 1915); WO 25/3548 (Embarkation Returns Abroad for Home Jan – Mar 1916); WO 95/2083 (War Diary 57th Infantry Brigade HQ 1915 – 1917); WO 95/2085 (War Diary 8th Bn Gloucestershire Reg't Apr – Dec 1916); WO 95/2264/4 (War Diary for 2nd Bn Gloucestershire Reg't 1914 – 1915); WO 95/4302 (War Diary for 39th Infantry Bde & 7th Bn Gloucestershire Reg't 1915 - 1916); WO 329/2707 & WO 339/1147(Gloucestershire Reg't Medal Rolls).

- Newspapers: North Wilts Herald, various dates 1914 & 1915; Swindon Advertiser, various dates 1907 & 1914; Wilts & Glos Standard, various dates 1914, 1915, 1917 & 1920.

- Oxford English Reference Dictionary. OUP 1996.

- Soldiers of Gloucestershire, Museum of the Gloucestershire Regiment. Undated Manuscript extract of 'The Lone Soldier - Reflections from the 1914-1918 War.'

- Spencer, William. 'Army Service Records of the First World War'. Public Record Office 2001.

- Steele, Nigel and Hart, Peter. 'Defeat at Gallipoli.' Macmillan 1994.

- Swindon Medical Officer of Health – Annual Report 1908. Published by Swindon Borough Council

- Thacker, Fred S. 'The Stripling Thames'. Thacker 1909.

- Thornicroft, Nick. 'Gloucestershire and North Bristol Soldiers on the Somme'. Tempus Publishing Ltd 2007.

- Timms, Peter. 'Swindon Works 1930 -1960.' Amberley Publishing 2014.

- Tomkins, Richard and Sheldon, Peter. 'Swindon and the GWR'. Alan Sutton 1990.

- Verey, David and Brooks, Alan. 'Gloucestershire: The Cotswolds.' Buildings of England Series. Penguin Books 1970.

- Waller, Ian. 'My Ancestor was an Agricultural Labourer.' Society of Genealogists 2010.

- Websites: www.1914-1918.com; www.ancestry.co.uk; www.armyservicenumbersblogspot.co.uk; www.britishnewspaperarchive.co.uk; www.findmypast.co.uk; www.firstworldwar.com; www.mangoldhurling.co.uk;

www.parliament.uk; www.qaranc.co.uk;
www.thisismoney.co.uk; www.wikipedia.org;
www.wirksworth.org.uk

- Westlake, Ray. 'British Regiments at Gallipoli.' Leo Cooper 1996.

- Westlake, Ray. 'Kitchener's Army.' Spellmount Ltd 1998.

- Whiyates, R. Ed. 'Artillery and Trench Mortar Memories.' N & M Press in facsimile edition 2004.

- Williams, Alfred. 'Life in a Railway Factory'. Originally published 1915. Republished by Alan Sutton 1984.

- Wilson HW & Hammerton JA (Ed) 'The Great War. The Standard History of the All-Europe Conflict'. Amalgamated Press 1919

- Wiltshire & Swindon History Centre: File Refs: A1 255/150 – A1 355/419 (Various Electoral Registers for the Parishes of Crudwell, Oaksey, Poole Keynes & Swindon covering the years 1905-1965); File Refs 667/1/1-5 Various documents including the copy will of Henry Poole, 1722; OS maps for the Poole Keynes locality 1900 (Wiltshire Sheets 4/6, 4/9 & 4/10); Wiltshire Monthly Intelligencer, July 2014.

- Wyrall, Everard. 'The Nineteenth Division 1914-1918'. Originally published 1932, republished by Naval & Military Press 2009.

ND - #0443 - 270225 - C12 - 229/152/14 - PB - 9781861515308 - Matt Lamination